W9-CUP-243

Julia Loggins is a fountain of wisdom and humility. Her work is born out of authentic inquiry, struggle and success. She is a pioneer and a seasoned professional, and her unwavering commitment to HEALTH in mind, spirit and body is awe inspiring. Julia speaks and writes from a wellspring of empirical knowledge and a heart of gold."

Dr. Jennifer Freed,
Co-founder of The Academy of the Healing Arts

"Dare to Detoxify!" is a handy guidebook to the deep cleansing process. For those who are taking full responsibility for their health, the book provides a detailed and highly personal manual for detoxification. Julia's personal stories make the book an exceptionally easy read."

Dr. Gay Hendricks, Author,
"Conscious Loving," "The Corporate Mystic" and "The Big Leap"

Julia engages the reader immediately with her prolific & passionate style of intimately sharing her own past health challenges, so that the reader feels a compassionate connection & a renewed sense of optimism about "How to Achieve Optimal Health & Invigorating Energy" with an exciting & adventurous strategy of "how to get there" by applying specific principles of detoxification that guarantee amazing results!

Dr. Janet Hranicky
Hranicky Cancer Program, The American Health Institute
Los Angeles, California

"This book is a treasure – easy to read, humorous, full of life-saving information. The step-by-step directions are invaluable! Anyone who reads it will be encouraged and inspired to eat well and live well…"

Betty Hatch,
Founder, The Self Esteem Council of Santa Barbara
Santa Barbara, California

1

The information presented in this book is in no way intended as medical advice or a substitute for medical counseling. It is intended only to provide the opinions and ideas of the author. It is sold with the understanding that the author is not engaged in rendering medical, health or any other kind of professional services in this book. The reader should consult his or her medical doctor, or any other competent professional, before adopting any of the suggestions in this book, or drawing inferences from it. The author disclaims any responsibility for any liability, loss or risk, personal or otherwise, which is incurred as a consequence, directly or indirectly, of the use and application of the contents of this book.

Please consult your physician before beginning this program, and use all the information the author suggests in conjunction with the guidance and care of your physician. Your physician should be aware of all medical conditions that you may have, as well as medications and supplements you are taking.

All client's names have been changed to protect privacy, and all stories are composites of clients seen in The Clinic.

Cover credits:

Cover Design by Budi Saputra—*Omini Design,* budidana@yahoo.com
Photography by Deb Halberstadt, Halfcity Productions
Makeup by Tru Beauty, Patricia Guererra
Hair by Silver Scissors, Stella Sapios

Published by Vibrant Health Publishing:

120 1/2 W. Mission, Santa Barbara, CA 93101
Phone: 805.563.0062, Website: www.DaretoDetoxify.com
Publishing Coach: Deborah S. Nelson, www.PublishingCoach.org

All Rights Reserved.

Copyright © 2012 by the author of this book, Julia Loggins. The author retains sole copyright to her contributions to this book. No part of this book may be reproduced or used in any form without permission from the publisher. The original purchaser is hereby granted permission to print the pages for personal use. Otherwise, copies of this book may NOT be transmitted, stored, or recorded in any form without written permission from the publisher, Julia Loggins, who will prosecute any violations of copyright law, including e-mail attachments or any other means.

Dare To Detoxify!

BY JULIA LOGGINS,
Certified Colon Hydrotherapist

For Luke and Hana

And to the memory of two bold spirits,

Dr. Ann Wigmore and Niravi Payne

TABLE OF CONTENTS

ACKNOWLEDGEMENTS

First, I thank my clients, who have courageously shared their journey with me; and in their willingness to open and reveal what they considered most toxic in their lives, have taught me so much about trust, acceptance and letting go.

I want to thank Allen and Anita Mills, whose work has changed thousands of lives, and whose friendship I cherish. I am so grateful for the opportunity to share you both with the world!

My daily thanks to my partner at The Clinic, Wesley Roe....for your huge and pioneering spirit; you have made our workspace a sanctuary, truly a "safe place to heal."

To Andrea Cagan, the best editor in the world...and a treasured friend. You are a magician.

To Deborah Nelson, publishing coach and mentor par excellence, thank you for assisting me in taking this project out into the world.

Thank you, my patient children, Luke and Hana, who shared me for nine months with the computer, while I wrote this book. Luke, thank you for your belief in me, your humor, and your high ideals, which both inspire and humble me. And thank you for your company in the kitchen! Hana, thank you for your comraderie, your passionate love of life, for having a beautiful song to hum, and for the dream we share of riding horses on the beach together at sunset...and for always reminding me, "Carpe diem!"

To my step-children, Crosby and Brooke, Cody and Bella, thank you for drinking wheatgrass when you were sick, and other strange things that came from having a weird step-mother; and thank you for the big arms you've put around your unique family.

To my sister, Susan, who inspired and guided this project with love, tenacity and vision – thank you! With all the places you contribute in your life, you always find the time to be there for me.

To my nephews, Zev, Ari, Noah, and my brother-in-law, Paul, thank you for teaching me what "showing up" as a family really means.
To my mom, Jacqueline Cooper, thank you for your love and support of me and this book, and for the enormous grace you've brought to all the transitions in your life.

To Kenny, thank you for teaching all of your children, and me, by your example and constant, caring and creative presence, that art is not confined to one project, or one genre, but is the willingness to continually re-invent one's life, to take risks, and that we're never too old to dream.

To Dr. Jan Hranicky and Dr. Michael Galitzer, thank you for your friendship and medical support, and your vision of creating a cutting edge integrative health center that supports the heart as well as the body; Dr's Brian and Anna Marie Clement, of Hippocrates Health Institute, for forty years of fierce dedication to the belief that anyone can heal;

Dr. Jim Blechman, whose kindness and creativity re-defines what doctoring is – for the motto, "Whatever works!"

To dearest friends, Adela Barcia, Dr. Kathleen Boisen, Clovis and Grady, Angelique and Michael Millette, Diane Murphy, Peter Pomeranze, Josette Troxler, Amy and Josh Wilson, thank you for sharing this wild ride with me....

To Cointa, Lino and Miguel Reveles Trujillo, for being our second family...

To Paul....thank you for finding me again; for sanctuary, and for the fire.

FOREWORD

God Bless Julia Loggins. She has written a wonderful book, "Dare To Detoxify," teaching us how to apply the essential elements of detoxification in order to optimize our health.

It takes a brave woman to reveal how the life threatening events of her childhood shaped her destiny, and led her on the journey to regain her health. Julia's battle with environmental illness took years to overcome, at a time when medicine, both allopathic and integrative, had very little to offer. That she overcame so much is a tribute to her instincts, tenacity, and wisdom.

Toxins are those physical substances which produce energetic imbalances in an individual. These imbalances can result in physical, emotional and mental symptoms. We are constantly exposed to toxins every day. There are two types of toxins, exogenous and endogenous. Exogenous toxins are present in the outside environment, whereas endogenous toxins are produced as a result of imbalances in our metabolism. Major exogenous toxins which affect us are:

1) Tap water
2) Smog and petrochemicals
3) Coffee, tobacco, alcohol, sugar, food preservatives
4) Pesticides
5) Heavy metals: mercury, aluminum, lead, cadmium
6) Viruses: Epstein-Barr, influenza, cytomegalovirus, herpes, HIV
7) Bacteria: streptococcus, staphylococcus, salmonella
   (food poisoning)
8) Parasites
9) Prescription medication
10) Over the counter medication

Endogenous toxins are produced as a result of compromised digestion and inefficient metabolism. They result from pancreatic digestive enzyme deficiency, poor eating habits, and wrong food combinations. Examples are candida and elevated blood levels of uric acid.

Julia shows us how to optimize our digestion. She gives us the necessary tools as to how to shop, where to shop, food combining, and the necessary supplements – HCL, pancreatic enzymes, and probiotics - that are necessary for great GI function.

Illness begins in the digestive tract, where 70% of the lymphatic vessels of the body reside. The lymph is essential for absorption of fats from the small intestine, for its immune stimulating effect through the Peyers Patches, and for its key role in detoxification. Julia teaches us about the value of lymph massage in moving the lymph, the importance of deep breathing in stimulating lymph flow, and the value of exercises such as a rebounder and jumping rope in further mobilizing the lymphatic system. She then shows us how to be kind to our liver, for don't forget that its first four letters are live.

After optimizing our lymph and liver, the next step is to dump those toxins out through the colon. Let us remember that the surface area of the intestines is 200 square meters, while that of the entire skin is 2 square meters. Thus even though one has a daily bowel movement, the colon may not be that healthy. Thus, the value of colonics and enemas.

Julia brilliantly covers the area of acid/alkaline. She shows us which foods and supplements to take in order to alkalinize our bodies. More importantly, she shows us what not to do. Her 21-day detox diet is very effective, and easy to implement. She takes us step-by-step through this process, utilizing juicing as a key component. Most of us are novices in the area of juicing. Julia makes it easy to learn.

Dare to Detoxify is a book for everyone seeking to optimize their body, and slow the aging process. If you want to get healthy, go see Julia Loggins.

Michael Galitzer, M.D.
Director, American Health Institute

INTRODUCTION

This book is borne out of the experience I gained saving my own life, and thirty five years of practice supporting others to do the same. Although I believe our diamond natures are refined by polishing (bruising and bumping!) — most of us have plenty of character already. We have busy lives and a lot on our plates. But without consistent good health, we struggle – physically, emotionally, spiritually and even, financially. Most of us know someone challenged by chronic or even catastrophic illness or disease. You may wonder what, if anything, can be done to prevent or minimize the same fate. We know our world is toxic, and yet, it's our home, and we aren't going anywhere!

We don't want to live in fear, either. Every day, my clients ask me what they can to do boost their immune system, re-vitalize their constitution and clean out the cobwebs of their attitude and their anatomy so that they can be as healthy as they can possibly be, with excellent energy and a positive picture of their present and future. Whether at home or traveling, they want to have crystal clear thinking, and the freedom to work hard and play hard in pain-free bodies. They also want to look and feel beautiful. One of the best tools to this end is, detoxification.

Detoxification means something different to everyone. To one person it means getting sober, in reference to drugs and alcohol; and to another, it refers to fasting, or going without food, for a period of days to achieve a physical or spiritual cleansing. In this book, detoxification is understood to be the basic recognition and release of what doesn't serve us – whether it's sugar, junk food or even, a bad relationship. In our clinic, we've learned from our clients that it's hard to confront and change a part of our life that's not working if our minds and bodies are hurting, exhausted, constipated and polluted. And, with our environment challenged as it is, it's impossible to escape pollution! We can, however, do something about the permanent damage pollution can do to our physiology.

This book is a roadmap to simple, successful detoxification. In it are all the tools that I share with my clients, everyday. Detoxification can be approached step by step, in your own home. Though some of the concepts outlined here may be unfamiliar, in time and practice, they will become comfortable, and integrate into the flow of your life and diet. We all have an awareness of what is good for us, even if it takes some practice to tune in and discover what it is.

If you become overwhelmed, with the information or the practice, take a break. Many of us have been trained to force ourselves when we're frustrated or fatigued; instead, please take a walk or go to the movies. We are initiating a new way of being, just by allowing ourselves to let go of needless suffering and pain in our lives, and the sources of that pain – in fact, just by acknowledging that we are in pain! That lesson is not learned overnight. And it's easier to do with a companion; if you can enlist a friend in the detox journey, all the better. Dare someone you love to get healthy with you!

In this book, you will meet some spectacular practitioners who practice modalities that support cleansing and detox. Check the website, daretodetoxify.com, for a referral listing of detox support practitioners in your area. My hope and intention is that the tools in this book, the stories I share and the people you'll meet will ignite your desire and nurture your ability to feel better than you've felt in years.

It's amazing what we can accomplish when we feel good! That is my wish for you…to have the boundless, unencumbered energy you had when you were a kid, and the effortless excitement for each and every day that went with it.

When I teach, I always begin and end my seminars with a prayer. And thus, we are beginning.

> *To Spirit, to all the energy in the universe,*
> *The pulse of life inside my body, the shooting stars in my heart,*
> *The blueprint of vitality and radical energy, passion and pleasure*
> *That I carry in my soul…*
> *Please fill me with the courage to let go of all that no longer*
> *serves me. I thank the thoughts, the foods, the substances and*
> *Even the friends who allowed me to survive the*
> *Trauma and chaos of my past.*
> *I ask for help in remembering who I am,*
> *Who I was born to be;*
> *Who I will smile easily at in the mirror.*
> *I ask for help in dumping the toxicity in my life,*
> *In whatever form it takes,*
> *And most of all, I ask for support in opening to*
> *Strong, consistent good health, happiness and my unique purpose*
> *As I move with power and grace and*
> *Without hesitation, into my beautiful, daring and delicious life.*

PART ONE
Who We Are

CHAPTER ONE
Our Clinic

Joanne was fifteen minutes early, as she stood in the doorway to our clinic. The wind was blowing so hard that the palm trees were nearly bending in half as leaves flew through the atmosphere. It was raining hard – an unusual weather pattern for Santa Barbara. But it was a perfect day to meet Joanne, since she was somewhat of a hurricane herself – a dynamic, sparkling type A personality, 45 years old, with a mahogany sweep of hair and expressive brown eyes. Wearing black boots and wrapped up in a wool fedora, she gave me a huge smile and thrust out her hand to take mine.

"I'm Joanne, great to meet ya!" she said in a booming voice, as I ushered her inside. She took off her wet wrap, and I invited her to sit down. At first glance, one might assume that this take-charge career woman was at our clinic because she'd heard a colonic would help her function better, think more clearly, and flatten her stomach (all of which are true.) But when we began our consultation, her real story emerged as she spoke without hesitation.

"I've been to hell and back," she literally exploded before I asked her a single question. "I drank non-stop for 15 years until I nearly died.

Because of my drinking, I got into two car accidents and I've had three major back operations. Then I got sober, met my husband, and had my son.

"I'm here now," she continued, "because my dad died of colon cancer and my digestion is so bad, it's scaring me. I go to the bathroom twice a week, and then only if I take herbs. I hate taking laxatives. And talk about heartburn! The acid in my stomach is like an inferno, no matter what I eat. I've tried everything. And I have no energy. It's a miracle I get through a day. But I own a post-production studio in L A, and there's no down time in my life."

I nodded. Years ago, I was in a life-threatening situation that I reversed by utilizing the methods in this book. In fact, this book was born out of what other practitioners and I learned from decades of experience with our own and our clients' detoxification processes. Some of us had life threatening illnesses. Some of us were just sick and tired of not having the natural energy, enthusiasm and passion that comes from a healthy body which also supports a peaceful and happy mind.

And so, over the course of my practice, I'd heard many versions of what Joanne was telling me now. It was thirty years ago when my partner, Wesley Roe, started what he called *The Clinic for Drugless Therapy* in Santa Barbara, CA. I joined forces with him in 2003 after having had my own private practice for many years. Both Wesley and I have been students of detoxification for decades, and each of our clinic practitioners (none of us are medical doctors or scientists), have healed ourselves of life-threatening illnesses without the use of drugs or narcotics. Hence, the name of the clinic.

Between Wes and me, we see about fifty people a week, and the main complaints are: Constipation, allergies, fatigue, depression, food and substance addictions, immune disorders, skin disorders, Irritable Bowel Syndrome (IBS), ulcers, colitis, migraines, PMS, breast congestion, lymph congestion, infertility, asthma and acne. Hearing what Joanne had to say was not new or unfamiliar, as she carried on without taking a breath.

"My GP," she spoke with contempt in her voice, "said there's nothing wrong with me. Nothing. I had a colonoscopy and I had to drink that awful salt solution for two days straight to flush out my system enough for them to see anything! But now they say nothing's wrong. Come on! I'm not stupid. And let me tell you, without my anti-depressants, I'm a train wreck. Pretty sad. Always have been, I think. Probably why I drank.

"Of course, everyone in my family drank. Funny, I was off anti-depressants for a couple of years and I seemed to do okay until I had my son. I guess even good things can push me over the edge cause as much as I love my son, I can't lose these last 20 baby pounds, even when I starve myself. I mean, I thought I knew how to lose weight cause I used to be a dancer. But now I don't have what you'd call a slow metabolism. I have a non-existent metabolism.

"Please," she practically begged me. "Do you have any answers for me? I'd do anything! I swear I'd fuck a fish in a barrel if I could get some relief! Well, I would if I had even one ounce of energy left."

She was making me breathless as I gently interrupted her diatribe. "Joanne, slow down," I said. "Just listen, because I have some answers for you."

She stopped and stared at me, frustrated but also expectant. After all, her doctors had told her she was fine. It must have been great relief that someone believed she was in pain, and was about to tell her the truth for a change.

"The trouble here," I said once I had her full attention, "is that your colon is so impacted, it's signaling your metabolism to slow down to a crawl so you won't flood your body with toxins! That's what impacted colons do in order to save our lives and our organs. It's why your metabolism can't be sped up with diet or exercise alone. You have to clean yourself out first. The drugs you had to take for your surgeries are still hanging around in your liver, making your adrenals work overtime."

I checked to make sure Joanne was still listening as I went on, "Your body is so acidic, you aren't making digestive enzymes so your food isn't digesting. Instead, it's getting dumped into your intestines without being absorbed. It's no wonder you don't have any energy!"

I explained to her that 95% of serotonin, the all important neurotransmitter that regulates and elevates our moods, is manufactured in our gut. Because Joanne didn't have the correct acid to alkaline balance to make serotonin, she was depressed. "Have you had digestive problems your whole life?"

"Absolutely," she said. "Since I was a kid."

"We inherit these susceptibilities," I told her, "but they're not life sentences. You already proved that by getting sober. You don't have to suffer for the rest of your life! It's simple, really. I'll just tell you what worked for me and for so many other people."

"I'm all ears," Joanne said. "I HAVE HAD IT UP TO HERE!"

I could see that she meant it, as we embarked on a cleansing program that I knew would help her tremendously. I felt confident, not only because Joanne was so committed to reversing her bad health, but

20

also because I felt secure that about 80% of our clients experience a permanent change in their conditions after a series of colonics. There is nothing like success to bolster trust and enthusiasm. In Joanne's case, since she was willing to go on a healthy detox diet with plenty of fresh vegetables, while limiting her intake of white flour, carbonated beverages and processed foods, I believed she would have great results – and she did.

I ran into her recently and she had tons of energy; she moves her bowels naturally every day (a miracle for her), and she just bought a new home. We all know how stressful moving can be, but Joanne was stable in her mood and she had cut her anti-depressants in half, on her doctor's recommendation. Best of all, she reported much more patience with her children and no anxiety attacks, which she'd been having regularly before she embarked on our program. Finally, with the loss of ten pounds and a new, steady exercise routine, Joanne was glowing through and through.

How about you? Is any part of Joanne's story your story? Do you wish you could quiet the embarrassing belching, the acidity and the pain in your gut? Have you ever fantasized that the large amount of gas you pass on a daily basis could run your car, or wondered why that last fifteen pounds feels cemented to your thighs even though you're exercising hard? If you are overwhelmed by a random deluge of confusing and conflicting information about digestion and detoxification, read on. This book is for you, born from decades of experience with my clients and my own detoxification processes. In fact, all the action steps in this book are designed with the knowledge that when we act courageously in our own behalf, not only will our body heal, but so will our hearts and minds. By doing whatever it takes to be healthy, we earn our own self-respect. And, believe it or not, that has a lot to do with good digestion.

In our clinic, we have seen clients in serious discomfort or even danger successfully transform their sluggish, slow-to-metabolize, often overweight, uncomfortable and congested bodies into lean and mean toxin-fighting machines. Those of us trained in the art and science of cleansing and detoxification, assist ourselves and others along a hero's journey of liberation from chronic pain, acidity that causes serious disease, and the emotional suffering that disconnects us from our hearts and eventually shuts down our immune systems. It takes a healthy person to be creative, joyful and productive as we pay the rent, reinvent our careers, heal our relationships, and stay sober – goals that are much easier to meet when our hearts and minds are free from pain, fear and toxicity.

Whether it's physical pain like migraines or colitis, or emotional challenges like addictions and depression, people are suffering. One of the reasons is that our environment is taxing our bodies in a way they weren't built to handle. As a result, the simple detoxification tools that I learned to facilitate the healing of my own serious illnesses are now required to keep all our clients healthy and vibrant, regardless of how robust their constitutions are, or were. It isn't enough to simply take a multi-vitamin and avoid fast food.

Whether you're strong and healthy and you want to stay that way, or if you're facing a life challenging illness, you may want to use our program in conjunction with whatever traditional or alternative support you are receiving from your doctor or practitioner. However you choose to use the information provided here, my mission is to present to you, in the simplest of terms, a tried and true program that can help you reduce toxicity, restore your natural acid/alkaline balance and allow your digestive system to heal.

When this happens, your entire physiology re-aligns. Your blood sugar balances, your energy increases and remains consistent, your moods lift, and you can end the cycle of difficult symptoms like constipation, heartburn, bladder and yeast infections, allergies, and auto-immune disorders that traditional medicine may treat but really cannot cure. Once you achieve a balance, you are freed from feeling like a frustrated two-year-old who wants to put everything in his or her mouth like fast food, sugar, fat, and caffeine, just to feel better, even for a minute.

After thirty five years as a health practitioner, I can say with certainty that detoxification of the colon and lymph has proven to be a key principal in returning to radical health those whose suffering was not alleviated by any other means. After all, the body's desire and natural state is to be healthy. Here is my story.

CHAPTER TWO
My Story

I never dreamed of becoming the "Queen of Detox" when I grew up. What teenage girl lies in bed at night thinking how cool it would be to pump impacted poop out of other peoples' colons for a living? Certainly not me. In my future dreams, I was something sexy like a ballet dancer or an Olympic equestrienne. But since I was a child of the sixties, I also dreamed of being a revolutionary of some sort – someone who could change the world.

Sounds like high hopes, right? Well, before you imagine me as the most altruistic child that ever lived, the truth is that I had selfish reasons, personal ones, that made me want to change the world – you see, the world was killing me. Literally. I was afflicted with an illness that was virtually unknown in the sixties: Environmental Allergies. No one, including myself, understood that in essence, I was allergic to the twentieth century – to the pollutants that made the blue sky look brown and to the remarkable new chemical additives that allowed a loaf of bread to last for a month without going stale. Most significantly, I was allergic to the plethora of steroids and epinephrine drugs that the doctors prescribed for me to suppress my daily asthma attacks.

By the time I turned six, besides my ongoing battle with life-threatening asthma, I had rheumatoid arthritis, migraine headaches, constant acute bladder and kidney infections, bleeding ulcers, diverticulitis and colitis. At six years old! My mom reminded me that my first words were, "My stomach hurts!" I really don't remember my stomach ever *not* hurting. I just thought it was an unpleasant part of life that everyone had to endure.

Throughout my childhood, I lost my hair twice due to severe drug reactions. No wonder I was rebellious, angry and confused, since my appearance was being compromised, and it was a struggle for me to think clearly. Today a physician would likely diagnose me with Attention Deficit Disorder (ADD), but back then, those three letters, ADD, had not yet been strung together to define a physiological condition. I was in and out of hospitals often during my childhood, and the simple act of concentrating in life and in school was a daunting challenge for me because (as I would learn later) my asthma medication was literally shredding my stomach and intestines. As a result, I absorbed very few nutrients, I had recurring insomnia and my blood sugar was always soaring and crashing.

Along with my environmental allergies, I was unfortunate to be among the shockingly large numbers of teenagers who experience sexual abuse and rape. The personal details of my abuse are irrelevant to this book, but the numbers are staggering, as our current research tells us that one in four people (men and women) in the United States will experience some form of sexual violence. I dealt with it like so many others – I unconsciously dissociated or "left my body," a survival and coping mechanism I discovered at an early age to numb my unmanageable feelings. But that kind of disconnect deteriorates the immune system from the inside out, as it promotes a level of acidity that can lead to serious illnesses like cancer and diabetes. When we disconnect from our bodies to such a large degree, we are also separated from our instincts, the intuitive parts of ourselves that allow us to identify and choose what is right for us in the most challenging of situations.

So at 17, I was losing my hair, I was bloated from steroids and pain-killers and I had monthly anaphylactic allergic reactions which resulted in rip-roaring, late-night trips down the freeway to the Emergency Room. The resulting brain fog and confusion from both the emotional and physical toxins in my system caused me so much depression, I really didn't need the doctors to tell me that I was dying. (Although more than one of them did.) My allergic reactions were becoming more frequent and severe, and survival seemed like nothing more than an optimist's hallucination. What had happened to my dreams of becoming a ballet dancer or an Olympic equestrienne? In my current state of disease and discomfort, how would I ever become a revolutionary and change the world? It was impossible to imagine doing much of anything from an intensive care unit.

I remember thinking to myself when I was a rebellious and wild 18-year-old that if I ran out of asthma medication and the drug store happened to be closed, that I would die. I wasn't free. I was "owned" by my disease and my dis-ease. And I had been since I was five years old. It wasn't until I met Dr. Robert Pottenger – whose family pioneered the research regarding food and environmental allergies – that I began figuratively to see the light at the end of the tunnel. Well, I suppose I actually *did* see the light at the end of the tunnel – quite literally – three times when I had near-death experiences from allergic reactions to food and drugs. But gratefully, the last one occurred in Dr. Pottenger's office during some routine food allergy testing.

I remember I was reeling that day from having been told by another doctor that I would never be able to have children. (I eventually birthed two, so what did they know?) But apparently, the so-called experts had agreed that my constitution was just too weak to carry a child to term. I had always wanted children, so I was in a deep depression, and I remember sitting in a chair, getting my arm poked with tiny specks of tree and flower antigens, when I was suddenly watching the scene from about three feet above my body. I learned later that I was having an anaphylactic reaction, an allergic response which can cause death almost instantly. But while it was occurring, I floated in the ethers, calmly watching my body, while Dr. Pottenger anxiously pumped my body full of adrenaline as he waited for the paramedics to arrive.

Still floating above the action, I watched several EMTs hooking up electrodes to my chest when I felt a powerful THUD on my heart. Then I heard a voice that said in a rather matter-of-fact tone, "You are not ready to die. You will heal. You have work to do and you will do it in this life, in this body, on this earth. And you are not alone."

When the voice quieted down, I felt peace. I remember that the most – being pain free and feeling calm and at ease. When I looked over at Dr. Pottenger, I figured he had to be an angel if such entities existed, because by simply looking in his eyes, I felt loved, seen, and accepted, which lifted me out of my depression. He was nothing short of a miracle in my life, as I felt relieved and bathed in his grace. Part of me had wanted to make my exit from this world, to abandon the compromised and complicated body that so often failed me, humiliated me and made me feel so different from the other kids who reveled in jumping rope and eating candy. They were free from the inhalers that had become my life line and the orthopedic shoes I was forced to wear. All I wanted was to be like them.

But thank God for a few renegade professionals like Dr. Pottenger, who recognized what was tearing me apart. He was smart enough to discover that a combination of the drugs, the foods that were toxic to me, and the toxins in my environment were not only affecting my body. They were also affecting my mind. He was the only adult in my life at that time who understood that my severe mood swings were not attributable to what others labeled as my having a "damaged personality."

After the giant THUD that occurred from the paramedics pumping my chest, my heart was jump-started by the drugs they were using and I came back into my body, into that room in Dr. Pottenger's office. I can't say that I miraculously healed right then and there and was able to get up and walk away. In fact, I was admitted to the hospital and spent three days and nights there, recovering from my severe allergic reaction. But something had shifted inside of me. Although I was at a loss to articulate what actually had happened, I never had another near-death experience. And I trusted, absolutely for the first time, that I was not alone.

As time went on, I would learn about yet another component of my health riddle. It seems that psychological stress was compromising my body as much as the environmental toxins. Maybe even more. Here, I must nod to the brilliance of Carl Simonton, M.D., a pioneer in the field of psycho-neuro-immunology. This genius doctor posited the theory that our thoughts either create and sustain, or depress and disintegrate our immune systems. In other words, he suggested (rightly so) that when we feel happy, safe and at peace, we are likely to be in good health. On the other hand, when we're unhappy, threatened, or frustrated, we are much more likely to become ill. I guess you could say that along with my heart, my gut instincts were re-ignited that day in Dr. Pottenger's office.

When my first detox was over, Dr. Pottenger told my parents and me that he had a goal for me to be drug- and asthma-free. My parents seemed skeptical. After all, I had been suffering with severe symptoms for most of my life. But the doctor explained to them that I was having recurrent anaphylactic seizures because my immune system was almost non-functional. In this weakened state, even a miniscule exposure to an allergen was life-threatening for me. In other words, the very drugs I was taking to save my life combined with the toxins in my food and my environment were causing my body to degenerate. I had to get cleaned out in order to save my life. Once I removed the toxins from my system, he assured us, I could heal my digestion and the over-acidic condition that was causing my ulcers, colitis, and rheumatoid arthritis.

When I saw Dr. Pottenger get out his prescription pad, I was a bit confused. He had just made it clear that drugs were my problem. But instead of writing me a prescription for steroids, Percocet, Darvon or any of the other eleven different pills I was taking daily, he wrote me a prescription for a purely fresh, organic diet, without sugar, wheat, dairy or any other toxic food that was hurting me.

It was limiting to say the least. For the next two years, there were about eight foods that I could eat because they would not hurt me. But the doctor reassured me that when I had finally flushed all the drugs and toxins from my system and allowed my immune system to heal, my organs would regenerate, my stomach would stop bleeding, and my allergies would clear up. I chose to believe him since he was the first person who had given me any hope for as long as I could remember.

During my two year cleanse, I recall sitting down to dinner with a group of new friends and saying no to the bread, cheese, pasta, and desert. A woman sitting beside me said, "How can you stand that? If I couldn't eat whatever I wanted, I'd rather be dead!"

"Really?" I said. "You'd rather be dead? You'd rather feel like someone was pouring gasoline in your gut every time you ate, and lighting a fuse? You would choose that over eating a clean diet?"

Apparently, not everyone felt the way I did when I ate these things. They didn't have to shoot adrenaline into their thigh twenty minutes after eating a piece of cheese, which would definitely impact someone's food choices. We are all human, after all, and we generally do only what we have to do. If we can get away with something, we try. I can't tell you how many times I pretended not to be allergic to cigarette smoke so I could be like my 20-something peers who all met for a drink and a smoke at a local bar after work. I so wanted to be like everyone else, but after a half hour of indulgence, I would leave the bar wheezing and coughing. Then, it would take me two full days to recover and a month later, I would do it all over again.

I finally learned that no one was watching whether I drank and smoked along with everyone else. Nobody cared. It was the demons in my head telling me that if I couldn't swig with the best of them, no one would want to put up with me. The truth is that no one cared if I was doing coffee enemas instead of drinking cappuccinos. And if they did care, I came to realize that he or she was not much of a friend; or possibly, they had bigger demons than I did.

Back in 1987, I was very much in my healing process, living at The Hippocrates Health Institute, when African-American comedian/activist Dick Gregory spoke at Harvard. A vegan as well as a fiery and fierce advocate of natural health, Dick Gregory told us that what we ate and how healthy we were defined whether we we're free or not. This was a bold statement in front of a mainly black audience, during a time when "soul food" like collard greens and fried chicken, defined ethnic pride.

Dick Gregory knew what he was up against, when in a soft voice that was almost a whisper, he told us that were all enslaved by our addiction to food and chemicals, all of which numb our sensitivity, our ability to think, feel, react and respond. How could we be free, he asked us, if our sugar Jones was giving us diabetes? If our loyalty to fried foods was causing heart disease? How could we see ourselves as warriors, as creators of our own lives, if our minds were foggy from drugs and toxic food? This man was passionate that the most revolutionary thing a human being could do was to get healthy and to support those they loved in doing the same.

I left that lecture feeling inspired about the change I was making. I may not have grown up to be a ballet dancer or an Olympic equestrienne, but I did get to be a revolutionary after all. Now when I think back to 1963, I realize that although I was the only one on the school bus with asthma attacks from the gassy fumes, and although I was the only one who broke out in hives when I ate anything sprayed, waxed or processed, these toxins were affecting us all. I was just the canary in the coal mine back then, but these days, there are many canaries. For example, when my step-son had his sixth birthday party (that was more than two decades ago), five out of twelve parents handed me an inhaler in case their child needed it.

Today, helping others in the same boat forms the foundation of our work in the clinic. It is important to realize that none of us invented the techniques and practices that we present in our clinic and that I am presenting in this book. In fact, all of our methods have been around for the last hundred years. I was amazed to find out that Dr. Herbert Shelton, the father of the concept of food combining which we will discuss later, was popular with the early movie stars. Mae West, herself, credited the practice of colonics for her flawless skin, while other luminaries were adherent to a book called *Enzyme Nutrition* by Dr. Roy Howell, who educated the general public about supplementing their diet with digestive enzymes.

In this sense, there is nothing new under the sun that we do in our clinic. But we have the unique opportunity to share our practices and techniques daily with people who are suffering with everything from asthma to IBS to polycystic breasts. The best reward is watching our clients become symptom-free after they clean their guts, restore their digestion, and go on to maintain a healthy acid/alkaline balance.

Dare To Detoxify!

CHAPTER THREE
Our Program Is Born

No two people have been more important to me in my work than Allen and Anita Mills, founders of the Santa Barbara Center for Lymphatic Health. We have not only been referring clients to each other for years, we also have enthusiastically been each other's clients. Allen, one of the most compassionate and grounded men I've ever met, is a brilliant health practitioner and educator. His intellect is always guided by his heart. Anita, his wife and office manager, is a visionary who sees living on the cutting edge as simple common sense.

I'd heard about lymph therapy for decades and underwent a treatment or two, but I didn't feel much of a shift in my health – until I met Allen and underwent his treatment program in April of 2006. It was my good fortune to run into him, and now that I have had the privilege of working with a large number of his clients on colon care, I have come to understand that properly executed, lymph therapy is one of the most potent healing modalities that exists.

I recall one brisk winter afternoon when Allen, Anita, and I were having tea in the garden of their cozy home in Santa Barbara. As we chatted and shared our stories, we had an epiphany: Throughout years of problem-solving our client's quandaries and listening to what worked for them (what it actually took to get well and where one could "cut corners"), we had developed an effective protocol. Our evolving program designed for healing digestive complaints and systemic acidity had been very successful for all of us, but we realized that we had never committed it to paper. When we acknowledged that we had a cohesive, accessible and "digestible" protocol that could help more people help themselves than Allen and I could ever see in a month, or even a year, we decided it was time to let the cat out of the bag! So here it is, in this book.

Thinking back to when we first met, I quickly discovered that Allen and Anita became proficient in lymphatic therapy for exactly the same reason that I learned everything I could about detoxification: to save their lives, or, to be more precise, to save Anita's life.

Anita Mills is one of my heroes, not just because she was the inspiration for her husband, Allen, to discover lymph therapy. Not just because her husband has become one of the country's most prominent lmphatic health practitioners and teachers. And not just because she refused to succumb to fear and become another mastectomy statistic. I admire these things greatly in Anita, but she is one of my heroes because her commitment to her healing is consistent with how she has lived her entire 61 years, an example to anyone who wants to heal and become the best of who they can be: happy, at peace, doing what they were put on this earth to do, in love, and in the company of devoted friends and family. What's the point of getting healthy if you aren't living your heart's desire?

From the moment I met Anita, I could see that she was a woman on a mission to motivate those around her to listen to their instincts and to act on them. Of course she is human and she gets lost and distracted sometimes, but ultimately, she listens to her inner voice and her soul when she feels herself straying from the healthy direction she believes life is meant to be lived. She doesn't call herself a feminist because she doesn't like labels, but I see her as an example of feminine empowerment and strength, as she dares others to find the same qualities in themselves. She is not a vain woman; she doesn't much care what other people think, so when she had breast congestion that caused her intolerable pain for years on end, she refused a biopsy and the possibility of surgery. She simply said, "No," because she believed she would find a better way to heal – even though the way had not yet appeared.

She stuck to her decision, kept doing research, stayed open to possibility, and in 1993, an answer appeared. Anita had three sessions with a lymph therapist when her breast congestion began to dissipate. This was a powerful discovery for her, since her husband, Allen, was studying lymph therapy at the time. When he observed what was happening to his wife after only three sessions, he completely dedicated himself to studying this brilliant healing modality.

Allen soon attended a seminar led by a man named Skye David, MPT, a physical therapist, who had studied with lymphatic pioneer, Dr. Emil Vodder. Back in 1936, Dr. Vodder was the first physician to develop a lymphatic drainage technique. He presented his findings at the World's Fair in Paris, and later, Skye David developed the "lymphstar," an electrical instrument that works by the dissociation of interstitial proteins via ionization. Using light and sound to de-ionize trapped proteins that are creating inflammation and congestion, this anti-inflammatory device breaks the bond between the protein molecules, which get stuck together and need to get separated gently with the lymphatic technique, a subtle movement that does not resemble regular massage. Going too deep, one can actually make the congestion worse. That's why a person who has severe inflammation and gets a deep tissue massage may feel better for a little while, but then worse as time goes on. By the way, I love getting a massage – it's a wonderful technique. But it doesn't take the place of lymphatic drainage. They are two dramatically different things.

Lymphatic drainage, quite popular in today's world, allows the lymph to drain without stimulating blood flow. While ultrasound therapy may give some temporary relief to an inflamed area, the inflammation will most likely return because it does not address the source of the problem like lymphatic drainage does. With Vodder's lymphatic drainage technique, the lymph flows out of the body, taking a load of toxins with it, and is then replaced by fresh fluid, as the blood continues to flow freely.

Allen went on to study in the US at the Vodder School under the tutelage of the woman who ran the original clinic in Austria. His work with her led to the development of the therapy he now uses in his clinic. Something that began with his desire to help others, has developed into a deep understanding of how under-valued and under-respected the lymph system is in our healing journeys. According to Skye David, in our current mode of Western medicine, the lymphatic system is often seen as damaged and the nodes are ultimately removed, instead of healing them which would be a far better way to address this kind of problem.

Allen told me, "Lymph nodes, when they are doing their jobs of collecting cancer cells, are removed when they have cancer in them. But that is what a lymph node is supposed to do: collect mutated and aberrant cells. Without them, we'd all be riddled with disease!"

Today, everything that Allen, Anita and I have learned, we are compelled to share with anyone who truly wants to reclaim their health and their instinctual sense of self that accompanies that. As long as we all contribute what we know to free each other from the misconceptions of disease and toxicity, no one has to reinvent the wheel.

It is a great comfort to know that we are not alone, because anyone who embarks on a detoxification journey knows how humbling it can be. And yet, it inevitably opens our hearts and minds like nothing else. A good example is when I lived in the Boston brownstone of Hippocrates Health Institute for two years, from 1982-4, studying under Dr. Ann Wigmore, a brilliant medical savant from Germany. Dr. Wigmore believed that God gave us illnesses just to get our attention and give us a chance to re-invent ourselves, and she is the best example of her own beliefs.

I will never forget how she would run down the stairs of her four story mansion into the living room each Sunday afternoon, to greet her new "guests," mostly critically ill patients who came to the institute to live and study for a week or two. Some had undergone surgeries and were left with a few less organs than they originally had. Coming from all the over country, it was amazing that they even survived the trip to Boston, but they had nowhere else to go. For them, this was the end of the line. Remember, it was the 80's and alternative health was truly *alternative!* Hippocrates Health Institute was offering then, as it does now, a truly viable protocol for healing catastrophic illness, even if most Americans had never heard of it.

These patients would arrive with their medical files in hand – detailed exposes of their deteriorating bodies, often with the foreboding words, "six to twelve months to live" typed under "prognosis." I recall Dr. Ann grabbing one of those medical files in her hands, and staring intently into the eyes of its owner, her own eyes twinkling. She was almost levitating with excitement, the dappled beet juice on her cheeks that she used as makeup adding to her unique appearance. Barely 4'10", Dr. Wigmore spoke in a high pitched, thickly accented voice.

You can only imagine what these folks were thinking when she said to them, "This is the best day of your life!! You're here. And you have nothing left to lose, except everything you have been taught to believe about yourself, about healing, and about the cause and cure of disease. You will get well if you believe you can. I do. I know it. I know that the body is God's temple and He wants us to be healthy and happy, and eat foods in their natural form." She meant every word from the bottom of her heart.

"If you're ready to let go of all that is toxic in your life – bad food, a job you hate – healing is possible," she would say. "When we are at the end of our rope, we are really willing to let go and re-create our lives. Here, you will get in touch with what is poisoning you, and let it go. You will be well."

Dr. Wigmore and so many others have illuminated my journey that began with my near-death experience at 17. At 28, by the time I'd graduated from the Hippocrates Health Institute's Health Educators Course, I had studied nutrition, detoxification, living foods and the mind/body connection. Through trial and error, I had experimented with dozens of alternative health modalities, always on the lookout for the diet and supplementation program that was right for me, a long and expensive journey. I often imagine that If I'd known the simple tools that are outlined in this book when I started, I would be typing these pages from the private yacht I bought with all the money I spent on things that didn't work!!

But it's all about the journey, right? I'm happy to say that I learned something from everything I tried, and the way I live and teach now is a mosaic of many different protocols that I tried and either accepted or rejected over the years. After all, life is all about change … so let's make it change for the better.

PART TWO

THE THREE D'S OF DETOXIFICATION

CHAPTER FOUR
Why Detoxify?

We detoxify the body so it can do exactly what it designed to do – eliminate hazardous waste so our physical body can heal and vibrate with energy. But as spectacular as our bodies seem to be (and they are pretty spectacular), they have their limitations. They can only digest or eliminate what happened to be on this earth at the time our ancient ancestors were hunting wildebeests and collecting berries.

Obviously that doesn't include diet soft drinks, fruits and vegetables sprayed with pesticides, paint thinner, artificial sweeteners like aspartame or sleeping pills like Ambien. The two billion pounds of pesticides that are dumped on America's farmlands each year are foreign agents to our bodies. Can you imagine what Hippocrates, known as the father of Western medicine, would have thought about the medical challenges for anyone living in a world as polluted as ours? It did not occur to the ancients that every single person living in our modern world would need to incorporate a consistent system of detox just to thrive and survive. Even today, nothing in our physiology recognizes these pharmaceutical phenomena as food, and therefore, we have no ability to eliminate them. In other words, we can't poop or pee them out because they don't even register as food within our systems.

As a result of ingesting so much that is foreign and toxic, our bodies try their hardest to save our lives by shuffling the toxins we eat, breathe and absorb through our skin into our lymph system, our liver, our colon and our reproductive organs. When this happens, we become exhausted and out of balance, each in our own personal way. For example, some of us get anxious, some of us get depressed, and some of us just get fat. Over time, more serious consequences arise. We might get cancer. We might get diabetes. According to the Merck Manual (the physician's pharmaceutical bible), ninety percent of us will develop some type of colon disease in our lifetime.

Have you ever told someone that you just don't feel like yourself? Or maybe it's been so long since you felt good, you think, *THIS IS MYSELF!* Yikes!

When you catch yourself thinking in those terms, once you become aware of acid foods, acid rain, overcooked food, microwaves, and all the rest of it, you need to recognize that the poison is winning. It is messing with your emotional well-being, because every threat to your physical health is also a threat to your emotional health.

In simple terms, every toxin that is harmful to your body is also harmful to your mind. I have found over many years of working in detox, that even when people show very few physical signs of toxic poisoning, they can still be depressed, despairing, or even suicidal. Many adults and children who may not show tangible signs of physical distress, just can't seem to stay away from drugs and alcohol. Even after completing rehab, these individuals still struggle. The trouble is that although they may have achieved sobriety, the drugs they ingested for years are still hanging around in their intestines because they were never eliminated.

When old drug substances remain stuck in the mucoid plaque in the intestines, similar to the way plaque builds up on your teeth, your body must work overtime in order to function in such a constant state of acidity. The liver gets hit the hardest, and as the body tries to gradually release some of the residual substance in tiny amounts into the blood stream and lymph, it only creates a stronger desire in you to use that substance again. If you have ever tried to clean out, get off drugs, and failed, you know what I mean. It may seem like the devil lives in your body and has total control over you.

From what I have seen time and again, however, I know that healing is possible. After all, I have healed myself and have watched countless others do the same with the tools in this book, the very tools that you are about to learn to help you fight back. Do you know what your devil looks like? These creatures are masters at disguise, but we can break through by realizing that most diseases are caused by toxicity and acidity.

The following list are some common symptoms with toxicity as their source that may be dramatically improved by a detoxification diet:

Acne
Asthma
Allergies
Anxiety
Arthritis
ADD or ADHD
Autoimmune disorders
Bloating, gas and belching
Chronic Fatigue
Chronic infections
Colitis
Constipation
Depression
Diabetes

Diarrhea
Hypoglycemia
Digestive problems
Fibromyalgia
Mood swings
Hay fever
Headaches
Hormonal imbalances
Infertility
IBS
Migraines
Muscle pains and spasms
Obesity
Skin rashes
Spastic colon

If you are plagued by any of these, please read on. There are ways to recognize, flush out and eliminate for good each of the symptoms on the list. It all comes down to detoxification and the three D's:

- Digest
- Drain
- Dump

Today's disease statistics are staggering. Colon cancer has become the number one cancer threat in America, while breast congestion, if left untreated, can lead to cancer. But we can't control every factor in our environmental landscape, so what do we do? We can't undo our genetics either, or the fact that some of us had so many antibiotics as kids, we thought they were one of the Four Food Groups. There are things we can do, however, to make our bodies as happy and disease-resistant as possible, such as: go alkaline, detox regularly, and become warriors for our own well-being.

In our current world, practicing the simple techniques of detoxification are absolutely imperative to living the healthiest, happiest life possible! Who among us is not affected by our compromised environment or by the fact that most of our food is packaged and processed. While some products that boast "organic" are often grown in less than vibrant soil, every aspect of our lives, bodies and minds are effected by electro-magnetic pollution, low air quality, a lack of water purity, the chemicals we touch and taste, and the low value of our daily nutrition.

With the environment in its current condition, along with our stress levels being as elevated as they are, sooner rather than later, most of us will experience a highly uncomfortable, inconvenient, and expensive physical or emotional condition we never imagined would happen to us. And believe me, if you'd rather be dead than change your lifestyle, your diet, or do a coffee enema and detox twice a year, well – you're going to make a lot of morticians rich and happy!

When a new client who has been ill for a long time comes into our clinic, we don't sugarcoat what they are going to have to do to get well. We remind them that if they have been seriously ill or have been struggling with addiction for a long time, there is no quick fix. Healing will happen, but isn't going to happen overnight. Keep in mind that detoxification means everything toxic that went in, has to come out, and a cleansing crisis can occur which may be temporarily uncomfortable. Yes, we are supposed to feel better when we're doing everything "right" to get better. But sometimes there are headaches and lack of energy when the body is using all its fuel to flush toxins. If you have had a long exposure to environmental toxins or ingestion of medications, the healing period takes time and it will require patience. You may feel worse before you feel better, but what's the alternative?

No one wants to feel like crap all the time, and have to take endless bottles of pills in the hope of feeling better. No one wants to adjust to the limitations in the toxic body and mind as if that is what life was meant to me. Life is meant for living, and with our current economical and physical challenges, we need all the emotional strength we can muster. We want our minds to be sharp, which will make the concepts of self-care easier to embrace.

The best encouragement I can give you is the fact that considering my dubious health history, I haven't had asthma, ulcers or migraines in 38 years. I attribute this to my dedication to detoxifying as well as to some brilliant doctors and health practitioners, from Dr. Robert Pottenger to Dr. Ann Wigmore of Hippocrates Health Institute, and from Dr. Ernest Pecci of the Hoffman-Process to Niravi Payne of the Whole Life Institute.

Speaking of Niravi Payne, my two gorgeous teen-agers are proof that it is possible to beat the grimmest of prognoses. It was Niravi Payne who pioneered the mind/body link in infertility, and whose work allowed me to heal the belief I could not have kids, even after three miscarriages. She taught me that I needed to put up my dukes and fight, rather than cave in with self-doubt and fear. She taught me to celebrate the motto, "I deserve to be healthy, goddamnit!" I can still see her in my mind's eye, at age 85, in her pink jumpsuit with her fist in the air!

As we move on to the three D's, I ask you to keep in mind that the intention of this program is to give you the tools that will allow your digestion to heal by restoring your body's acid/alkaline balance. Only then can you can get on with your life, with your body humming happily along! I had to do every single piece of it to get well, to heal my digestion, and to have physical stamina. As I present the following information, I do so with determination and commitment, because I continue to live exactly what I am teaching.

CHAPTER FIVE:
The First D: Digestion

As important as the green juices are that we'll talk about later in this book, so are the positive and negative conversations that go on in our heads. We have spent years asking ourselves and our clients the big questions:

- How do you feel right now?
- If your stomach could talk, what would it say?
- How badly do you want to heal?
- How willing are you to change your lifestyle to experience the ecstatic energy you had as a kid?

Dr. Sidney MacDonald Baker, a practicing physician who has deeply researched the nutritional, biochemical, and environmental aspects of chronic illness in adults and children, says in his book, *Detoxification and Healing:*

- *If you are sitting on a tack, it takes a lot of aspirin to make it feel good.*
- *If you are sitting on two tacks, removing just one does not result in a 50 percent improvement.*

He also says,

- *You could substitute the word aspirin with psychotherapy, meditation, organic foods or vitamins and the rule still applies; the proper treatment for tack-sitting is tack removal. In particular, don't take medicine to cover up a symptom instead of looking for the cause.*

He goes on to tell us that the only two places in the body where our cells remain the same as the day we were born are in our brain and our immune system. In these two areas, our cells are undivided and unchanged and brain cells do not completely replace themselves soon after they die. As a society, we are conscious of protecting our brains, since we put on helmets when we cycle or schuss down the mountain on a pair of skis. But what do we consciously do to protect our precious immune systems? What do we do to make sure we are digesting our food?

Good digestion is critical to healing disease. When we don't digest our food, it becomes toxic, and toxicity creates inflammation, which the AMA recognized last year as the root cause of all diseases. In Europe, where that has been acknowledged for decades, lymph drainage and colonics are often part of national health care. It's all about supporting our ability to digest.

In our clinic, we define digestion as:

**What we ingest and absorb (thoughts as well as foods),
What we choose not to ingest or absorb,
And what we eliminate.**

In a perfectly healthy world, digestion should be as painless as breathing. And yet, for many of us, it clearly is not. Do you sometimes wonder why you feel lethargic and depressed? Have you ever noticed how much life sucks when your tummy hurts or your bowel is in spasm? The truth is that efficient digestion and maintaining an alkaline system makes everything else in the body work also. When it doesn't work, you are a walking time bomb for illness and disease, allergies, and even addictive behavior. If you're "starving" for nutrients, your brain kicks in and tells you it's okay to grab something to eat, *anything* that will make you feel good, happy, and safe. And when you're starving enough, you will grab just about anything.

So what if you used to eat poorly, but you have changed your ways? Of course that's better than continuing to poison yourself. But it's a popular myth that your body begins releasing junk, just because you have stopped shoving that junk into your mouth.

News release: Getting healthy and losing weight is not just about willpower!

The truth is that old poisons get stored in your liver, gall bladder, kidneys, colon, and the lymph system that runs through all your vital organs. These dangerous toxins end up in your bloodstream and lymph months or years after you may have stopped introducing them, wreaking havoc with your health and your emotions. It is only when the unhealthy substances that you so often crave have actually been flushed out of your system, that your desire for them are drastically reduced.

We call the absorption of the body's own waste "auto-intoxication," which makes you feel like you're sucking on the open end of a gas pipe. Are you nodding right now? If you're familiar with this terrible feeling, it will take creating some new habits to experience vitality and remain safe from the degenerative diseases that these poisons can create. Think about it. You do this automatically in other parts of your life. You get your car's engine oil changed regularly, you scrub the caked grease off the surfaces of your oven, and who among us expects our toilets to clean themselves? Would you go to a party at the end of the day without taking a shower first? Of course not. So why isn't it just as important to clean the inside of your body? It's actually more important because most pain and disease are caused and escalated by a buildup of toxicity and acidity.

Both high energy and emotional well-being are signs of health and vitality, and are necessary for us to thrive. So what are the main sources of the strength and liveliness we crave? Great digestion and elimination. Dr. Michael D. Gershon, M.D., in his groundbreaking book, *The Second Brain*, which he identifies as the bowel, says, "The ugly gut is more intellectual than the heart, and may have a greater capacity for feeling." He also says, "The brain in the bowel has to work right, or no one will have the luxury to think at all."

Did you know that there are close to one hundred million nerve endings in the small intestine, about the same number that are in the spine? This is why at least forty percent of visits to an internist are generated by gastrointestinal distress. Often people who visit the emergency room because they think they are having a heart attack, are really having a gas attack. Even a diagnosis of asthma can be traced back to mal-absorption or "leaky gut," a condition that occurs when undigested matter leaks from the bowel wall into the lymph and blood.

We talk about getting back in touch with your "gut instincts" because health and digestion are inextricably linked to our emotions and our ability to discern what's best for us, and then, mobilize. After all, what is digestion, but the decision concerning what stays and what goes? And we're not just talking about food here.

If we return for a moment to the last two elements in our definition of detoxification, (what we choose not to ingest or absorb and what we eliminate), we can see that along with reviewing what we should eat and drink to achieve pain-free digestion, we also need to focus on what we should *not* eat and drink. I'm referring to anything foreign or poisonous to the body which fall under various categories:

- Environmental toxins: substances such as pesticides and household chemicals.
- Internal toxins: waste products made by the normal bodily processes. These are the normal liquids and solids that we release through urination, defecation, perspiration and our regular inhaling and exhaling functions.
- External toxins: what we inhale and absorb through our lungs and our skin.
- Pharmaceutical toxins: substances such as drugs, caffeine and alcohol.
- Emotional toxins: repressed feelings and all types of emotional overload that arise from our day to day stress.

Each of the above toxins are devastating to the body. But the good news is that all varieties of toxins are easier to access when we commit to a detoxification program. Since ancient days, the sages knew that that the body needed special preparation for battle or to initiate a transformation, so they fasted on water and juices, allowing their bodies to release the toxins, to cleanse themselves, and thereby become healthier and stronger. As I mentioned earlier, detoxifying is hardly a new concept.

Today, even though the detoxification diet we suggest in our clinic (to be detailed later) is not as severe as a juice or water fast, the same principals apply. We eat certain foods and drink water and healthy liquids to remove the toxins that cloud our thinking and numb our emotions. My clients often remark that while they are on their detox programs, they not only feel better physically. They also gain mental perspective and clarity about their work, their relationships and their path and purpose in the world. It's hard to think about our purpose in the world when we can barely get out of bed in the morning due to brain fog, sluggish bowels and an acidic gut. Remember the old joke about men being led through life by their penises? In our clinic, we think a truer statement is that we are ALL led through life by our gut!

One has only to take a look at the changes in our environment in the last several decades to understand why we are having trouble digesting our food. We have gone from the land of "milk and honey" to the land of unsafe drinking water and genetically modified foods" (GMO). These are only a couple of reasons why detoxing needs to be a regular part of life, just like we automatically put on sun block to protect our skin from the harmful rays of the sun and we filter our water to protect our insides from unwanted chemicals.

Here are some statistics from the World Health Organization (WHO) that are extremely eye-opening:

- Over thirteen million deaths a year occur from environmentally-related diseases.
- One in three men and women between the ages of 25 and 40 are infertile.
- Nearly two billion pounds of chemicals are released every

year into the air. Almost six hundred million pounds of these chemicals are released on land through leaks or spills.

- Chemicals such that have that have been outlawed in the US, are used on fruits and vegetables in foreign countries, and exported to America's grocery stores.
- Over three thousand chemicals are added to our food supply in the US. Ten thousand other chemicals are used in food preservation, processing and storage.

When you review the list above, is it any wonder that we feel like crap? (Or, why we can't?!)

Of course there are "good chemicals" in our world as well, such as drugs like antibiotics that can save our lives when we get a staph infection or pneumonia. But even with antibiotics, there are dangers since they kill not only the bad bugs but the good ones, too. I'm talking about the natural flora manufactured in our intestines which protects us from Candida overgrowth, a yeast that can cause bloating, allergies, depression, and chronic bladder and yeast infections. Anesthetics – especially general anesthetics – which we need during a life-saving operation, will often cause constipation and depression. In those who struggle with chemical imbalances in the brain, such anesthetics can trigger emotional reactions that last for months. So even with the good comes the bad.

In her book, *Detox Strategy,* Brenda Watson, CNC, and Dr. Leonard Smith, M.D., tell us that more people die every year from reactions to prescription medications, medical procedures and treatments than from cancer or heart disease. The point is that whether it's the drugs we take over the counter or medications prescribed to us by our doctors, we are taxing our livers to the tipping point. Most of us don't need to go far to visit a toxic waste facility. We have become one.

This is why I am writing this book. As tough as the statistics are and as much of an uphill battle as it may seem, I'm here to tell you that it is possible to get these life-stealing toxins out of your bodies and balance your acid/alkaline levels. Even in an urban environment, it's absolutely possible to be strong and healthy without becoming a paranoid fanatic who walks around in a bubble. You simply need to detoxify and rebuild your digestion.

In our clinic, we are very grateful to the community of medical doctors, scientists and naturopaths who have researched and written extensively about this subject. Their work validates everything we live and teach! Given the pollution in our environment, and the stress of 21st century life, these techniques are no longer just for the seriously ill or the radical health enthusiast. They are useful for anyone who wants to live an optimal life.

The bottom line here is that you can heal yourself of toxicity and acidity because the concepts of cleansing are simple and straight-forward. Testing your pH (acid/alkaline) doesn't require a lab, a doctor or a hypodermic needle. All you need is a test strip you can buy at the drug or health food store. In this book, we will place the principals of detoxification, the tools and techniques of cleansing in your hands. Our goal is to make the information as easy to digest as the foods and supplements we recommend.

So what do Allen, Anita and I tell every one of our clients? We give them certain constants that have helped us in our lives – guidelines and cornerstones that will create good digestive health and alkalinity. Most importantly, we want our clients to believe that healing is possible, no matter how they feel, what they've been told, and how long they have struggled with pain and discomfort. The truth is that it's okay if you don't believe. If you've felt horrible for years, seen two dozen doctors and tried boatloads of diets and supplements that didn't work, why should you believe? Remember, I've been there, and all I can say to skeptics is, "Fake it til you make it." Being skeptical won't keep you from getting well, but not doing anything about your pain and suffering will definitely work against you.

CHAPTER SIX
The Second D—
Drain! Drain! Drain!

When you consider that the human body is made up of 75% water, it makes sense that lymphatic therapy would be the first course of action for anyone suffering from a serious illness. After all, we call the lymph the "river of life." Lymph therapy also makes sense for someone wanting to lose weight or increase energy. So why don't more people practice it? Although having clean lymph is as important to our overall health as having clean blood, it is often misunderstood and mostly ignored. We've all heard of lymph nodes, and most of us have had a doctor feel under our jaw when we were sick, but did you realize that lymph runs through every part of your body?

I am not a scientist or a medical doctor, but I will attempt to explain in layman's terms how the lymph works. Most of the water in your body exists in the form of "interstitial fluid," or lymph fluid. There is a continuous interchange between the body's trillion cells and your interstitial fluid, which is grayish in color. Food and oxygen are exchanged by the bodily fluids for waste products, and pressure from your arteries moves this fluid in and out of the cells to create a continuous circulation. As toxins are picked up by tiny lymphatic tubes or ducts, they are sent through the lymph vessels to be cleaned. You could say that it's always "laundry day" in your body as your cells are constantly being bathed and flushed, hydrated and oxygenated, fed and massaged.

If the toxins are *not* carried away, your living cells become compromised and even die, since their own waste can act as a poison. This is where things start to come apart. Or I should say, this is where *you* start to come apart, since the system of lymphatic ducts extends everywhere through your body, running alongside capillaries, arterioles and venules, which are all blood vessels.

Here is the most important thing to learn about the lymph: Unlike the blood system which is pumped by the heart, our lymphatic system has no pump in its vessels to push along the lymph fluid. Rather, the lymph depends upon the contraction of your muscles, the compression of your tissues from the outside, and gravity to move the fluids filled with waste to their main garbage dumps in the left and right sub-clavian veins.

At certain places along the lymphatic channels, lymph nodes collect toxins from cancerous growths and disease-producing bacteria. That's right, I said "Cancerous Growths." According to immunologist Lawrence Burton, PhD, of Nassau, the Bahamas, cancer and infection are *always* present in our bodies but our immunity protects us from actually contracting these diseases. In other words, we all carry cancer cells within our bodies but our lymph nodes prevent the spread of disease by keeping these cancer cells localized while keeping infections from spreading further. Can you see why the lymph is so important? It is literally saving our lives every single day.

You can feel swollen lymph nodes not only under your jaw but below the ear, below the collarbone, under your armpits (yes, men, too!), and in the crease between the thigh and pelvic area. You might feel some small bumps or lumps when you touch these areas, or a grittiness or a swelling from water retention, called edema. All these lumps and bumps are signals of blocked lymph nodes and vessels.

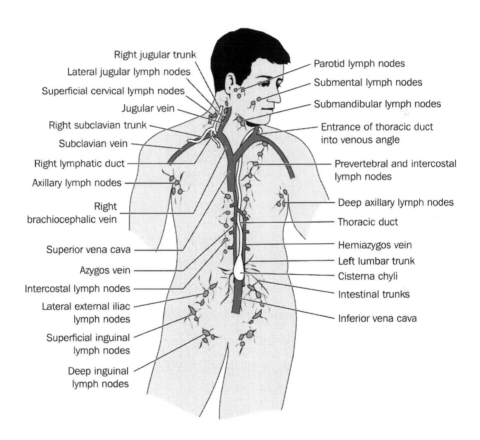

Dr. Arthur Guyton, M.D., professor and chairman of the Department of Physiology and Biophysics at the University of Mississippi School of Medicine, is an internationally famous expert on the lymph. His studies have shown us that a sluggish lymph can cause such degenerative diseases as cancer, heart attacks, strokes, diabetes, kidney failure, and chronic problems like headaches, depression, anxiety, and allergies. A sluggish lymph is usually the reason you catch every cold and flu that comes along. It can also cause varicose veins, hemorrhoids and blood clots. As you can see, there is a direct correlation between high energy, a strong immune system, and a highly functioning lymphatic system.

So what can a person do for themselves without paying a visit to a lymphatic therapist? *A Lot!* The lymph is not affected by our heart beat. Rather it moves due to outside stimulation. Therefore, exercise, particularly jumping, is integral to lymphatic health.

Here's a fun fact: Jumping on a trampoline or rebounder is one of the best known stimulators for the lymph.

These devices are not just for kids. Always remember that if you have kids or want to *act like* one, a large trampoline with a net around it, or a small rebounder (which fits easily into an office or bedroom) will provide a safe place for uninhibited jumping. If you spend ten minutes a day jumping up and down, that's a huge step in keeping your lymph moving and shaking and doing its job. The truth is that you don't even have to leave the house. Just bounce very gently up and down on your trampoline or rebounder; your feet don't even have to leave the mat, and that will force those fluids to move. Anyone can do it!

Another great tool to clean the lymph is called dry skin brushing. Of course, getting a lymph massage, or a series of lymph massages, is most effective, especially if you have a specific problem you want to address. But you can do this at home with a few simple instructions:

HOW TO DRY SKIN BRUSH

Use a long-handled brush with natural vegetable bristles, specifically made for skin brushing. Make sure you keep the brush dry, and not used for bathing.

On dry skin, use long, sweeping strokes – no rubbing or scrubbing, no back and forth motion; just gentle, sweeping motions toward the heart. The proper direction of skin brushing is essential to effective lymph flow. Brush up the arms towards the shoulders. Brush up the back towards the shoulders. Brush up the chest, starting around the belly button, up the center of the chest, and up and around the breast and up under the arms. Then brush the legs, starting with the soles of the feet; then up the lower leg to the knee; then upper leg to groin and groin to belly button.

Skin brushing is optimally effective if it's done twice a day, just prior to bathing. A complete skin brushing takes no more than five minutes!

The question is, why are we so resistant to the very techniques and processes that can heal us? Even I, someone who is open to new ways to feel better, was initially resistant. I had been seeing Allen's clients for colon therapy for years and had been blown away by their stories of success with lymphatic cleansing, before I experienced it for myself. It took my own crisis to engage me in an intimate and ongoing relationship to my own lymph system, and now I can only sing the praises of this powerfully effective therapy.

I was getting my yearly exam, a PAP smear and breast exam, from my nurse practitioner when she said, "Julia, you have cysts here I didn't feel last year. I know there isn't a history of breast cancer in your family, but I'm concerned. I'm sure it's nothing but we're going to keep an eye on this. I want to see you in three months to see if these cysts have grown. Don't worry. It's probably just hormones or stress."

In my world, "don't worry" are two of the most stress-producing words in the English language. The words "trust me" run a close second, at least when you hear them from your doctor. So I called Allen and made an appointment.

At my first lymphatic therapy session, Allen came into the room and began to check the lymph all over my body, as he ran his hands gently from the top of my head down to my toes. Once he had checked key lymphatic areas for suspect areas, he began to massage those lumpy places with subtle movements until they were smooth.

"I do feel congestion in your breasts," he told me, "and in your

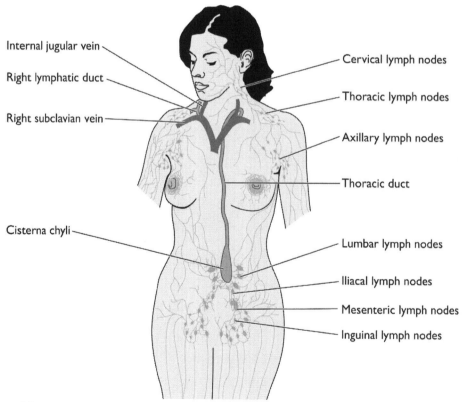

lungs, in your uterus . . in fact, everywhere!"

I was amazed at his sensitivities. It seems that a trained lymph practitioner knows simply by the feel of the skin, exactly how much congestion is there. Allen told me that inflammation or congestion has finally been recognized by the AMA as a major cause of disease, and lymph therapy is one of the most potent modalities to reduce that inflammation. Even for muscular congestion, lymphatic therapy is extremely effective.

Allen went on to tell me that two-thirds of our lymph is palpable, that it can be felt and seen right beneath the surface of the skin. That makes it possible to discern visible changes during the session as he works with the deep track that runs below what the fingers can palpate. Allen has explained that when someone is congested, he feels a grittiness right below the surface and he felt plenty of this in my body. I have to say that I was shocked at the time, because I'd been on an ultra-clean diet for 35 years, although I had never dealt with the lymph specifically.

He said calmly, "We can handle this." And I relaxed, feeling safe in his experienced hands. That's one thing of the things I appreciate most about Allen. As honest as he is about one's actual condition, he has absolute faith in the body and its ability to heal, a conviction that is so genuine, it's contagious.

I saw Allen for a series of lymph sessions, and at home, I dry skin brushed every day. In six months, my cysts were gone and I was ecstatic – until two summers ago when I got into a car accident. I was rear-ended, I sustained a whiplash and a concussion, and then, two months later, the cysts in my breasts came back. Now, I see that lymphatic therapy can be used as a restorative as well as a preventive. We have a saying at our clinic:

STRESS GOES TO THE BREASTS!

I did another series with Allen, I continued my dry skin brushing, and now, they're gone once again. It can be as simple as that. By the way, if the idea of a man or a woman touching your breasts during a massage freaks you out, you have my compassion, but ask yourself this: Are you more freaked out about getting a lymph massage or having your breasts cut off? After all, breast congestion can lead to breast cancer, just like uterine congestion can lead to uterine cancer and prostate congestion can lead to prostate cancer. So you choose. Gentle touching or brutal slicing?

"I made the discovery," Allen says, "that if the body is going to heal, it's the lymphatic system that's going to cart the junk out and detox the body. For detox, it comes down to the lymph system. No system works by itself. The lymph delivers these waste materials to the kidneys and liver to be eliminated from the body through the colon. (Do you see how colon therapy and lymphatic cleansing need each other?) It's extremely important that the colon is flushed after a lymph session, or the toxins will recycle and this can lead to some real problems. That's why people sometimes get sick after lymph treatments or any detoxifying treatment. They just aren't following up with colon cleansing. Colonics are key to the whole cycle of detox."

We all know we have a lymph system, but very few of know what it actually does. In fact, many people never consider it a key to health and healing but this is a big mistake. Think about how we treat our lymph system, as we overload it with too much salt, sugar, and fat. These toxic substances slow down the process because the lymph is already hard at work cleaning out environmental toxins.

The truth is that simply by triggering the body's lymphatic response, good lymph therapy can boost a person's immune system to the point that the body begins to operate the way it's supposed to, no matter what else is or was going on. It may not be the whole answer, but it's always, always part of the solution, because when the lymph system is strong and clean, the rest of the body can do its job. Think of the body as a miracle, which it is, and imagine that the lymph system is one of its miraculous tools. When you remove that tool – clog it up or cut it out – the body doesn't work optimally.

On the other hand, when you restore the body's capabilities to do its own work, healing is inevitable, because in the words of pop chanteuse Lady Gaga, "We were born this way." In fact, lymph therapy does not only release the congestion of a fibroid or cyst, it also releases decades-old scar tissue and adhesions.

My associates and I have seen clients who've suffered for years with internal adhesions from surgeries of all kinds: abdominal, thoracic, limbs and back. These kinds of adhesions cause immense pain and suffering, even if the surgery itself was life-saving. But most of these clients had given up on any kind of relief until lymph therapy allowed their internal scarring to heal. Were they ever surprised and gratified to find out that this kind of scarring was not permanent! They benefited the most from lymph therapy when they were post-op, since that is the best time to prevent such adhesions from forming. With some of our breast cancer survivors, we have found that with lymph therapy, the traditional post-op swelling and pain in shoulders and arms is avoided almost completely.

CHAPTER SEVEN:
The Third D–DUMP

I have saved the most controversial, most ridiculed, most disputed and one of the most effective healing modalities for last – the enema and colonic. I believe that enlightenment does begin with our asshole! In fact, in the clinic we have a cringe-worthy saying: YOUR SHIT IS MY BREAD AND BUTTER!

Colon cleansing and colonics have been a foundation of our program since we began. But just like most of us have so little understanding about our lymphatic system, the same is true of the colon. Even though colon cancer kills more Americans than any other form of cancer, colonics and enemas are like four-letter words to many people. It simply doesn't make sense then, that the subject of "poo" should be taboo unless you are under five years old.

Dr. Richard Schulze, one of the foremost authorities in the world on natural healing and herbal therapy, says in his book, *Detoxification*:

"EVERY American will develop some type of colon disease, polyp tumor or colon cancer in their lifetime. So it's high time we started talking about what's causing it, how to heal it and more importantly, how to prevent it."

69

When I first began my own serious detox program, I had nearly two decades of pharmaceutical drugs stored in my young body. Twice, I had been covered with boils for thirty days straight, I had migraines that would last for a week, and I could not think or concentrate for the life of me. After I began cleaning my colon, however, my skin cleared up, the migraines stopped, my colitis healed, I regained my clarity and my energy, and I lost the gas and bloating.

I have seen this happen with countless patients. Since colon cleansing can eliminate or drastically reduce most of the uncomfortable symptoms of toxicity and detoxification, such as headaches, nausea, constipation, diarrhea, rashes, hives and boils, anxiety, insomnia, migraines, gas, bloating, and "the shakes," I don't know how people do a cleansing without them! Actually, I do know how. They suffer unnecessarily.

Allen has had patients show up in such a severe state of detox after a lymph session, he doesn't simply *recommend* a colonic. He tells his patients that if they don't get one, they'll have to take a break from lymph therapy because their liver can't take any more toxicity.

Colonics, a primary component of the Gerson Therapy, one of the most successful alternative modalities for healing cancer and catastrophic illness, are not new. Enemas have been prescribed for a long list of ailments as far back as two thousand years in the *Manual of Discipline*, which is one of the books of the Dead Sea Scrolls. Enemas were also lyrically described in the *Essene Gospel of Peace.* In the Essene Gospels, colon cleansing was likened to a baptism, which cleansed the soul as well as the body. Colon cleansing therapies have always been a fundamental part of traditional yoga practices, as well as Taoist trainings. Hippocrates, himself, recognized as one of the founders of western medicine, practiced and prescribed enemas for his patients.

From the 1920's to the 1960's, the regular use of enemas was standard practice among European and American medical doctors in health spas and hospitals, for both children and adults. In 1910, Dr. Norman Walker established the *Laboratory of Nutritional Chemistry and Scientific Research* in New York, and began his extraordinary contributions to health and cleansing. Among his great discoveries was the value of fresh vegetable juices, and the development of the titrator juicer, which is still the Rolls Royce of juicers. His book, *Colon Health,* introduced his research on what he called "the keys to a vibrant life." It's only been since the dawn of the pharmaceutical age, post-Word War II, that colon cleansing, as well as other forms of alternative healing such as herbs, healing touch, homeopathy and nutrition, have not been recognized as a standard medical procedure. Well, the dog days are over!!

The greatest benefits of colon cleansing stems from removing the 5-20 or more pounds (yes, really!) of waste that is packed inside our colons. This is true, even if you're thin and in shape, and have a bowel movement every single day. I've given colonics to folks who were fasting – eating not one spoonful of food – and we watched old, putrefied fecal matter come out of their colons thirty days into their fast! These were healthy people, (or so they thought), doing a cleanse!

OK, let's have a little anatomy lesson here. The colon or large intestine is the last six feet of the digestive tract, located at the end of the small intestine. The ileocecal valve is the bridge between the small and large intestine. It leads to the beginning of the colon, called the cecum, which is about two inches below your right hipbone. It then goes counterclockwise to the ascending colon (going up your right side), your

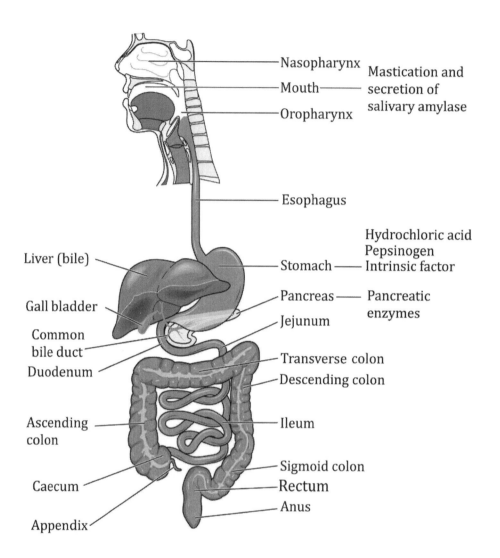

transverse colon (which goes across your tummy below your navel), your descending colon (down the left side), and the sigmoid colon (near the left hipbone). It ends at the rectum, which is about five inches long.

The colon is actually a muscle and if it lacks tone, then constipation is a given – not just constipation of waste in the rectum, but also in the entire large intestine. Did you know bad breath generally emanates from the private compost heap in your colon? That's why those mints don't always work! There's a great phrase that was taught to me years ago, "Machinery rusts and people rot!"

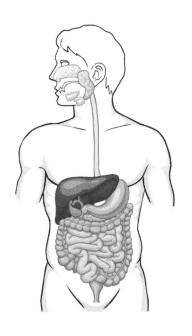

The colon has the ability to expand to such an extent that it either touches or is very close to every major organ in the human body except the brain. When it is packed with fecal matter, it can compress and crush all the organs it's touching – the lungs, the liver, the gallbladder, the pancreas, the kidneys, the adrenals, the uterus and the prostate. That's why a constipated colon can cause an infinite amount of health problems, just by its sheer mass! And that isn't even accounting for the toxins that are leaking out and poisoning the bloodstream.

The colon has pockets in it from beginning to end – bulbous pouches, really – and they contract similar to the movements of a snake. The ileocecal valve can be found an inch or two above the right hip, halfway between the hipbone and the navel. Its critical function is to automatically open and close so as to limit the reflux of colonic contents into the ileum. When pain is experienced here, it's often gas, which can hold the ileocecal valve open. This creates a wall of waste that backs up into the small intestine. Meant to be a one-way door, if fecal debris gets stuck in this area – as well as worms and parasites – there's trouble! Headaches, nausea, and even depression occur. Did you know that when actor John Wayne donated his body to science, forty pounds of waste was found in his large intestine? And the trophy goes to Elvis, who, at the time of his death, was reported to have had fifty pounds of waste in his colon!

The colon has very sensitive nerves and muscles that are meant to create wavelike motions – called *peristalsis* – to move the waste from the cecum out through the rectum. Besides peristalsis, the first half of the colon's job is to mulch and absorb through its walls, into the blood stream, whatever liquid nutrients the small intestine didn't collect. The blood vessels that line the colon walls carry this nutrition off to the liver for processing. Found near the ileocecal valve is a small, worm-like sack about three inches long which we know as the appendix. The

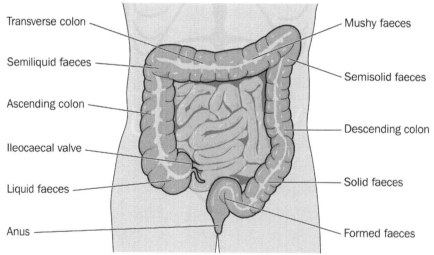

appendix is one of the lymphatic organs, and the primary job it has is to keep the ileocecal valve free of infection and inflammation. We all know what happens when this organ is toxic – appendicitis!

If the waste in the colon has putrefied and fermented, any nutritional liquid present that passes into the bloodstream is completely polluted. When this is the case, what would otherwise be used by the body as nutrition, becomes toxemia. This toxemia slows the metabolism to a mere gasp, which is why so many people on even the lowest calorie diets, doing high-powered exercise, still struggle to lose weight.

All of our food must pass through the 22 feet of the small intestine to our colon. But the Standard American diet is so sticky and full of chemicals, we do not assimilate and eliminate rapidly and very few of us have a bowel movement after each meal. If you have small children, check out the throne after they go. It will look like a Great Dane pooped in your toilet! This is a healthy functioning colon. But while the minimum a healthy body can eliminate is once a day, many of my clients who go once every three days would think they'd won the poop lottery if they eliminated once a day!

This slow, sticky journey of waste through the colon – a trip that can take days or weeks when it's supposed to take no more than 18 hours – causes not only putrefaction, but colon degeneration, due to the cells being bathed in toxic waste. This also causes spasms, infections, colitis and diverticulitis, which are incredibly painful diseases of the bowel. Did you know that low back pain is often associated with bowel distress and gas? When I was in my twenties, I had chronic low back pain until I discovered colon cleansing and food combining, which eliminated the gas that was causing it. I'm a proponent of chiropractic and gentle spinal manipulations, but no manipulation can do what colon cleansing does for chronic low back pain that is caused by gas and undigested food.

If your colon is a paralyzed, limp muscle, it is not going to push waste effectively out of your colon. When the colon is impacted, this leads to fecal encrustation of the colon walls, like a plaster cast, which prevents nutrition from being absorbed while it sends polluted waste straight into the bloodstream. Every day that the colon isn't eliminating completely, layer upon layer of dehydrated fecal matter is building up in the colon, like unpaid bills being smashed in a trash compactor! This is called writing a check that your tush can't cash! It's like toxic wallpaper decorating your colon with discomfort and disease, which will eventually find its way back into the bloodstream. Can you see how Toxemia is a disease we give to ourselves? (Read an amazing book on this subject: "Toxemia Explained," by Dr. John Tilden.)

Many of our clients suffer from toxemia, at one level or another. That's why they're sick! Their lymph is sluggish and their colon is packed like a sausage, even if they're vegetarian. But although most of the clients I see are aware that their colons need help, they have no idea what this toxic waste dump is doing to their liver and kidneys! That's why colon cleansing is so important for everyone, not just for people who have constipation.

When the blood becomes overburdened with toxic waste, the liver has to pick up the overload. Because the environmental toxins we deal with in day-to-day life are taxing our livers to the max already, this pushes them over the edge. Often, a client with a liver that is swollen and inflamed, will ask, "How did this happen? I don't smoke or drink or use drugs!" Yet every apple that's been sprayed with a chemical taxes the liver, as does every piece of chicken loaded with antibiotics and hormones. Now the kidneys are working overtime because the liver is dumping toxins south into them. Our kidneys are meant to purify bodily fluids and the waste from our natural, daily metabolism. They were not designed to take on heavy bowel toxins that should never have entered the body in the first place. Enter low back pain and kidney infections!

Next comes the bladder, sitting just in front of the last part of the intestine known as the sigmoid colon. When toxins leak into the bladder, inflammation, infection and chronic discomfort follow. Talk about leaking! Adult diapers are a billion dollar industry.

And now, the toxic burden is pushed into the lymph system, which is why lymph drainage is an integral part of detox. It is also why colon cleansing is integral to lymphatic health and the health of the entire body.

CHAPTER EIGHT:
Colonics

I once went to a convention of colon therapists and you've never met a happier group of people! We simply love our work because we get to see so many transformations. People who come in our doors feeling crappy, tired, achy, cranky, depressed and confused, leave feeling as if they're on cloud nine. That's the power of cleaning the colon. But the secret of colonics is not just that they cleanse the colon. They also release poison, which calms and soothes the entire nervous system – one of the best drugless highs you can ever have.

Many of my clients describe the feeling as being similar to the spiritual euphoria they experience after a vigorous yoga session. That's because it's completely safe and natural as we restore the body to its most natural state of being – toxin-free! So let me take you through the experience of having a colonic which will hopefully make you feel less afraid of something that is so freeing.

I now welcome you to *The Clinic for Drugless Therapy* in Santa Barbara, which I mentioned earlier in this book. Between me and my partner Wesley Roe, who started the clinic thirty years ago, we've been students of detoxification for 64 years. And I have to say, everyone should have a colon therapist and a partner like Wes. A master story teller with a witty sense of humor, a well-versed student of both psychology and physiology, Wes sometimes sings to his clients as they open to not only the physical, but also the emotional and spiritual journey of colon cleansing and detox.

When I walk into my waiting room to meet a colonic virgin, he or she is sometimes more nervous than if they were about to go up in the space shuttle! Occasionally, I'll have clients that need to be gently peeled off the walls. This is only natural because once they share their stories, it comes out that they are either abuse survivors, had horrific experiences with a grandmother forcing them to do an enema as a child, they were shamed for pooping in their pants, or they may be struggling with constipation so fierce that everything associated with elimination has a painful and scary tone to it. Colonics are healing for everyone, but most of all, for those who carry these challenging experiences and memories. We call our clinic, "a safe place to heal," because our most important job is to provide safety, confidentiality and trust during the release of toxins, both physical and emotional.

Our machine is state-of-the-art, and all our equipment is disposable so there is no chance for infection. As you lie on the massage table, face up and knees slightly bent, you gently insert a smooth, plastic tube into your rectum (called a proctoscope.) Yes, the term "tight-ass" is literal. The nerves around the rectum do affect the whole body, and when they're tight, you're uptight everywhere. So even the gentle insertion of the tube begins to relax the nerves in the entire body.

After insertion, which is extremely slow and soothing, you won't even feel this tube at all. You will only notice the feeling of warm water flowing in and out of your colon, in small amounts, as your colon therapist massages your tummy. We do this to work the water into the pockets and flexures of the colon, so that the old matter easily releases. It's not painful at all, though at first, it's an unfamiliar feeling to trust that the body will easily release waste in a lying-down position, without any effort. Always remember, colonics are gentle. Introducing water and fluid inside the colon is a completely natural thing. In fact, though the colon can easily hold two quarts of liquid while during a colonic, we introduce no more than 4-16 ounces at a time.

Although this is not always clear to people, our machine is *not* sucking the poop out of your colon! Your colon is doing 90% of the work, because this procedure is like taking your colon to the gym. In some cases, it's more like CPR! Clients who have used laxatives for years have very little muscle tone in their colons, so it's not uncommon for absolutely nothing to come out – and I mean nothing except the water we just put in – for an entire first colonic, which lasts about an hour. Hard to believe? If you want inspiration to change your diet forever, come spend the day with us and see what we get to see, because during a colonic, you can see everything that is coming out.

For us, it's the most fascinating movie in town, since we have seen worms, copper pennies, and hundreds of thousands of dollars worth of undigested vitamins and supplements flowing through the glass tube. When clients have been fasting before the colonic or have been using colon cleansing supplements that sweep the waste off the colon walls, we'll often see one to two feet long releases of impacted fecal matter. This is the waste that has been hanging around the colon for years.

Did you know that the colon is the center of release for early childhood trauma, as well as sexual abuse, and PTSD of all kinds? This is why clients sometimes get in touch with experiences or memories they have blocked for years. That is one of the great gifts of colon cleansing. Even without specific memories, verbal communication or intellectual processing, the release of toxins allows for awareness to light up certain areas, emotional and physical, that have remained hidden in the dark for years. Releasing the taboo in our culture around our poop empowers the colonic experience to help us integrate parts of ourselves we have long-ago separated from. And any time that happens, human consciousness, health and vitality take a giant leap forward.

Yet another great benefit of colonics is that they re-hydrate the gut. Some of our clients are so dehydrated, it's impossible to obtain a satisfying release during the session. When we see this, we recommend several treatments in close succession. That lets the client know that they must increase their fluid intake to increase the release and to make the treatment smoother and more comfortable. We can't stress enough the importance of hydration. Until you are regularly hydrated, you may not even realize that some of your distress comes from lack of water.

After a colonic, we advise our clients to drink plenty of water, take a probiotic to replace the bowel flora, and also to drink an electrolyte drink. Electrolytes, frequently ignored but incredibly beneficial supplements to add to your water, are not just for marathon runners. Electrolyte drinks which contain sodium and potassium salts, replenish the body's water after dehydration from exercise or excessive alcohol consumption, diarrhea, vomiting, or eating toxic foods. We recommend electrolyte packets such as Emergenc-Lite, that don't have added sugar. There are also electrolyte packets that don't have added vitamin C if you have a sensitive stomach.

When the first colonic is over, clients usually ask the question, "How many do I need to thoroughly clean my colon?" Generally, the answer is between 6 to 12. Will a dozen colonics completely clean all the waste out of a colon that has been abused or neglected for 50 years? Probably not. But it's a good start. Colon cleansing, lymph therapy and a detox diet are all procedures that we recommend doing yearly, to maintain optimal health.

LILLIANA

My client, Lilliana, had struggled with some form of addiction all her life, whether it was sugar, alcohol or pills. When she was forty, after a divorce and losing a job she loved, she checked herself into rehab and got clean. Healthy and proud of herself, she figured she would stay that way for the rest of her life.

But she had a chronic problem she couldn't seem to fix: insomnia. Lilliana tried everything natural she could find, determined to stay away from wine which had always relaxed her and helped her sleep. When she asked her doctor what to do, he told her that the occasional sleeping pill, Ambien specifically, was not habit forming and she could try it.

In the beginning it was like a miracle. One half a pill put her out for the whole night. She was ecstatic and got her prescription filled regularly with no questions from her doctor or her pharmacist. (It's amazing how many clients I see whose doctors don't question the refill prescriptions.) When she was invited by friends to Hawaii for her

42nd birthday, Lilliana was thrilled because she loved Hawaii so much. But she didn't bring her sleeping pills with her. This was not a conscious choice. She just forgot in the excitement of packing for this trip.

She was so active during the days, swimming in the ocean and walking along the white sand, for the first three nights, with the waves splashing outside her hotel window, she slept like a baby. But on the fourth night, she couldn't fall asleep. She couldn't sleep the next night either, and by the sixth night, she was sweating and shaking all night long as sleep eluded her.

She shook all the way back home on the plane, and after barely making the drive home from the airport, she crawled into bed, still shaking and began to vomit. She had no idea she was detoxing the sleeping pills, because she never realized she was addicted.

Lilliana must have had good angels watching over her and great gut instincts, because before she left on her trip to Hawaii, she had booked a colonic shortly after her return. When I met her in the waiting room of the clinic, instead of seeing the beautiful, polished blond I remembered from some months prior, Liliana looked like a cast member of *Survivor*. She had not slept for days, she had barely eaten, and the first thing she did was apologize for how she looked.

When she began to tell me her story, I found out that she had become addicted to sleeping pills and had spent the last few nights in hell – panic attacks, uncontrollable shaking, nausea and vomiting. When she did manage to close her eyes and doze off, she was in night terrors and hyperventilation.

"I've been through some tough stuff in this life, Julia," she told me, "but the last few nights were worse than anything I've ever experienced. I thought I was becoming psychotic, and I had no idea I was addicted to those damned pills. This is the worst head trip you can imagine. I'm finally starting to keep some food down after a few days, but I feel sick to my stomach all the time and my head is killing me."

She went on to tell me that she went to a medical center earlier that day, and the doctor there offered her Valium to calm her down and get rid of the shakes. "But dammit," she said, "I don't want any more pills."

Aware that she was dehydrated, I made Liliana an electrolyte drink and after she drank it, she felt a little better right away. We tested her pH and found that she measured 5.5. That was quite acidic; I wasn't a bit surprised, and I told her that eventually our goal was to achieve a pH of between 6.4-7.4.

When we started her colonic, she began to relax, and as the toxins started to leave her liver, her headache dulled and started to go away. She experienced waves of nausea throughout the colonic, which is normal when the liver is dumping bile, but by the time she left, she was nausea-free. I explained that although she had released a lot of bile in her first session, she was still in detox and it would take several more sessions to stabilize her.

I saw her twice that week, twice the next week, and by the fourth session, she looked like a different woman than the strung out Lilliana I'd met ten days before who could easily have been mistaken for a bag lady after a bender! After just four colonics, her pH was now close to alkaline, she was drinking liquid chlorophyll every day, and she was sleeping five hours in a row, substituting her sleeping pills for calcium magnesium, trace minerals and electrolytes. Two weeks later she was sleeping for six straight hours with no drugs.

"Man," she said to me, "I wish I'd seen you the first day I

stopped taking those pills. I wish I'd known I was hooked on sleeping pills, and that there was a way to get off them that didn't have to cause as much trauma as what I went through. I never want to go through that again. I want to really clean my liver out for good, from all the years of poison I've swallowed. It's a new day and it's time for a new body."

CHAPTER NINE:
Enemas

Enemas are self-administered colon cleanses. They can be done at home using water or infusions of aloe vera juice, wheatgrass, coffee, herbal teas such as chaparral or slippery elm, or essential oils, like chamomile. Enemas are really helpful to flush out the toxins which a detox initiates, so it an important process for everyone to know how to do.

People want to know if they can become dependant on enemas or colonics. The truth is that anyone can become dependant on anything. When I was living at Hippocrates Health Institute, I met a man who was addicted to oranges. He ate about 40 a day, so people can get addicted to all kinds of things. But the goal of colon cleansing is the opposite of addiction. It is about getting the colon's own peristalsis to work better, not to become dependant on anything, even herbs. After a course of treatment, our clients' colons work better than they have in their whole lives, because the impacted waste and putrefied gasses were keeping them from going to the bathroom. Recently, I had a client e-mail me a picture of a one and a half foot poop she had, *on her own*, after a lifetime of constipation, because she was so proud.

COFFEE ENEMAS

Coffee is a powerful, effective medicine when used as a rectal implant. We owe this discovery to Dr. Max Gerson, founder of the Gerson Therapy, who developed a technique for liver detoxification and reducing pain in the body by introducing coffee into the colon. In a story that Charlotte Gerson tells in her book about her father's work, the use of coffee for this purpose most likely dates back to the time of World War 1. Soldiers were sent back from the front lines, severely wounded, in need of surgery, and there was so little anesthetic available, they found a way to use coffee for this purpose. The nurses were used to giving enemas to the soldiers immediately following surgery, and the story goes that one day, a nurse decided to pour some coffee into her patient's enema. The pain relief was so profound, that this became a regular practice with surgical nurses.

In the 1920's, two medical professors had their interest aroused by these stories. Dr. O. A. Meyer and Professor Martin Heubner, M.D., of the German University of Goettingen's College of Medicine examined the effect of caffeine given rectally to cats. They discovered that the caffeine stimulated the cat's bile ducts to open, and they published their findings in the German medical literature. Dr. Gerson learned of this research, and it launched his study of coffee enemas.

This is how coffee works when it's introduced into the gut, as described in "*The Gerson Therapy*":

All of the body's blood passes through the liver every [few] minutes. The hemorrhoidal blood vessels dilate from exposure to the caffeine; in turn, the liver's portal veins dilate, too. Simultaneously, the bile ducts expand with blood, the bile flow increases, and the smooth muscles of these internal organs relax."

This process detoxifies the blood serum and also promotes peristalsis. The flushing of toxic bile is further affected by the body's enzymatic catalyst known as glutathione S-transference (GST.) The GST is increased in quantity in the small intestine by 700 percent, which is very beneficial to the body since this enzyme squelches free radicals. In 1990, Dr. Peter Lechner, M.D., while investigating Dr. Gerson's treatments, reported that GST blocks and detoxifies carcinogens among other things. He decided that the coffee enema had a very positive purpose: lowering serum toxins, literally cleaning the poisons out of fluids nourishing normal cells.

Simply put, coffee enemas (also referred to as coffee implants) dilute portal blood and bile. They counter inflammation in the gut and enhance the GST transference; they promote peristalsis. Because all the blood in the body passes through the liver every three minutes, this treatment represents a form of dialysis of blood across the gut wall. Coffee implants are phenomenal for people who are struggling with symptoms of drug withdrawal, because they pull the toxins right out of the blood stream. They can often eliminate a headache (or hangover) immediately, and are quite effective for migraine sufferers. When I was dealing with asthma attacks, coffee enemas would greatly reduce and often quiet the attack.

One of the most amazing things about coffee implants is that they calm the colon. Homeopathy often deals with opposites, and just like the homeopathic "coffea cruda" is given to calm the nerves, coffee enemas work the same way.

If you're caffeine sensitive however, try using chamomile tea or wheatgrass enemas rather than coffee. Although the caffeine in a coffee enema is rinsed out of the colon with clear water infusions so that there isn't any "buzz," it's still possible to absorb a small amount of caffeine through the colon. Dr. Gerson recommends retaining the coffee rectally for fifteen minutes for full effect (more about that in the next chapter), but we've found that it is a very effective liver cleanse when it's only retained for 2-5 minutes, which allows those who are caffeine sensitive to still avail themselves of its good medicine.

To make coffee for your enema, be sure to use organic coffee. Use one to two tablespoons of coffee and add it to two quarts of water; boil it, and then simmer it for 5-10 minutes. Strain it through a fine strainer, and cool or add ice to bring the liquid to body temperature. DO NOT USE REGULAR INSTANT COFFEE! Even organic instant coffee has acid, which is taxing for your body.

HOW TO DO AN ENEMA

I never travel without my enema bag, because an enema can provide immediate relief from an allergic reaction. It will also make you feel better if you have a headache, cold or the flu, and is one of the great tools of detoxification when a colonic isn't available. A note about shopping for an enema bag: Buy the kind with an open top because it's so much easier to pour the water in. You want to look for a two quart hot water bottle with attachments, and not the disposable enemas that are sold over the counter.

Until modern medicine taught us, erroneously, to take a pill for whatever ails us, enemas were one of the first tools anyone turned to when they were sick. It's common sense. Get the waste out, and whatever bug is traveling with it, and you'll feel better. Enemas are easy to do, so when my clients ask me exactly *how* to do them, this is what I tell them.

First, make your bathroom warm! Put on some nice music. You're going to be there a while, so create atmosphere. Get out the book you're reading and light an aromatherapy candle. This is a great time to listen to books on tape or that CD study course you thought you'd never have time for!

Put a large and preferably old towel on your bathroom floor. Get a couple of pillows for your head and put them at the end of the towel. You're going to hang the enema bag about 18 inches above your head, so the doorknob works great, and so does the shower door.

Apply plenty of herbal ointment, like calendula, or un-petroleum jelly to your rectum. Even Dr. Bronner's peppermint soap will do! Over-grease! Fill your enema bag with warm water which is body temperature or a little cooler. Lie on the floor, insert the end of the tube gently into your rectum and let out the clamp, which lets in a little bit of the water. If you can take in 8-16 ounces, that's good. You may feel an initial cramp and think, "Oh, I can't hold this! I've gotta go!" That's OK. Just sit on the toilet and let everything flush.

Repeat two to three times. Try to take a little more water each time. Breathe slowly and deeply. If you feel a little cramping, shut off the flow of water and breathe through the cramp. It may take a few bags of water to really get things moving!

When you're lying on the ground, slowly turn to the left, and then the right, for a few minutes each, massaging your belly, counter-clockwise. Start on the right, below your hip, and move across your tummy to the left, towards your splenic flexure, which is next to your spleen. Try to hold the water for at least five minutes, with your feet up against the wall or even in a modified shoulder stand, if you do yoga. If not, just put your feet up straight against the wall, propping your hips up a bit. Adding a towel or two under the hips helps. When a cramp comes and you know you're ready to flush, sit on the toilet, rubbing your belly, so all the water releases from the pockets in your colon that you have massaged the water into.

A cecum dump is when the water has gone up into the entire colon, all the way to the cecum, by the ileocecal valve, and the entire contents of the colon are flushed out at once. It's difficult to get what we call a "cecum dump" with an enema, but if you do enough bags of water and create a really complete release, you might! You will know if you do because it's hot, and you'll feel a peristaltic wave from your right side to your left. It's amazing! Like an orgasm, you don't wonder whether or not you've had one. And it's one of the great benefits of a colonic. But remember, whenever you need to alleviate detox symptoms and you can't get a colonic, enemas are great, even if you don't flush your colon all the way to the cecum.

Now that you have really flushed your colon, you can do an implant with coffee. Try to hold the coffee for 5-15 minutes, as long as you are not caffeine sensitive. (Even three minutes will help your liver flush.) You will need to follow this implant with three bags of pure water, to flush your colon and clean the caffeine out of your system. It's important to follow the last water flush with an implant.

An implant is a liquid such as wheatgrass or electrolytes which is inserted into the rectum, after a colonic or enema, to balance the metablolics in the colon. Take two ounces of wheatgrass, or two ounces of water infused with an electrolyte mix (one without sugar added), and insert that into your rectum with a baby ear syringe. It's the perfect syringe for the job! They are available at any drug store. Like your enema bag, it can be cleaned after each use, dried, and readied for your next session.

Once you get over the taboo connected to enemas, you will be amazed at how therapeutic they are. Just imagine. You can often get rid of a horrible headache or stomach ache in twenty minutes in your own home, without drugs! It's much healthier to give yourself an enema than it is to take a harsh laxative.

CHAPTER TEN:
The Santa Barbara 21-Day Detox Diet

Now that we have covered the three D's, I would like to present to you a three week detox diet plan designed to offer the tools that we give our clients at The Clinic. You have most likely surmised by now that it takes more than three weeks to detox your body from a lifetime of toxicity, so treat this regime as an educational experiment, a launching pad. It is just the beginning; but in three weeks, you'll feel so much better than you do now, I can guarantee there will be no going back!

Think about it. How many of us live consistently on clean diets that are completely free of white flour, sugar, fried foods, coffee or alcohol? Not many of us. So how do we not only exist, but thrive, in a world which has become a challenging biosphere? How do we avoid becoming a statistic of early cancer, diabetes, heart disease or depression?

The good news is that we can be pro-active rather than feeling like a time bomb for illness. And it doesn't require that we live a neurotic, paranoid life, deprived of pleasure, isolated and separated from all we have associated as delicious, comforting and celebratory.

None of us have to live as if the house is on fire. Instead we can arm ourselves with a fire extinguisher and get busy. I'm referring to putting into practice some tried and true strategies that can save your life. I know what they are because they saved mine. Just keep in mind that when we are cut, we heal. If we don't, we probably have a deep, systemic infection and a weakened immune system that may require an antibiotic or an herbal or homeopathic remedy. There are simply times when our body has been so taxed, it is no longer capable of responding to healing infection. But it is crucial to remember that the medication is not doing the healing! It is merely killing off enough of the infection so that our bodies can take over and do the job. That is what happens when we remove the toxins from our bodies and the best way to do this is to go on a detoxification diet.

Here, I am presenting a powerful detox diet that has helped me as well as countless patients in our clinic. As you read on, remember that nothing in this book is intended as professional medical advice or treatment. I am not a medical doctor and have no authority to prescribe any course of therapeutic or medical treatment. I am simply sharing what has worked for me and for so many others around me. As with all dietary and healing programs, please consult your doctor or health care professional before practicing or putting into use any of the information in this book. And please make your physician aware of the medications and supplements you are currently taking.

If your current medical practitioner doesn't believe in the holistic approach, however, and has no experience in supporting patients through the process of reclaiming their health through diet and detox, don't expect him or her to belt out a huge "Good for you. It's about time!" When a doctor once told me that the ideas I am presenting here were a load of bullshit, I told him that bulls had nothing to do with it.

"The shit I'm eliminating," I informed him, "is entirely my own!"

If you are faced with a serious health condition and take medication for it, I encourage you to look for a practitioner who is supportive, well-educated in detoxification, and able to monitor your blood work and whatever other tests you may need. The amount of medication you are required to take often changes as your body heals, and there are doctors available who are excellent guides along this journey. Look for someone trained in integrative medicine: the combination of conventional and alternative modalities, which is most definitely the medicine of the future. For reference, The American College for Advancement in Medicine is a group of doctors dedicated to practicing integrative medicine. Their website is referenced at the back of this book.

As I present this suggested diet, I want to make it clear that the goal of this program is to detoxify, alkalize and cleanse your body! Our bodies' perfect pH balance is 6.4, so between 6.4 and 7.4 is your goal. Do the ACID TEST every day! This is easy because pH strips are available at your local drug store.

After the first 21 days, by experimenting with the foods, supplements and the tools we'll share in the following chapters, you will be able to determine what affects your digestion badly and what you can get by with. You will learn what the occasional "party" foods are, what makes your body sing day to day, and what, if anything, simply spells disaster. Allen and Anita and I all have different lists. Everyone does. And our lists change as the cycles of our lives change.

21-day Detox Diet

You may have all you want of the following foods, which are all alkaline. Everything should be organic!

VEGETABLES: Leafy greens, sprouts, beets, broccoli, cabbage, carrots, cauliflower, celery, chard, collard, cucumbers, dandelions, dulce, edible flowers, eggplants, garlic, green beans, green peas, kale, kohlrabi, avocado, sweet potatoes

GOOD FATS: Avocado oil, coconut oil, flax seed oil, olive oil, omega 3-6-9 oil, UDO'S oil, borage oil, hemp oil

NUT MILKS: Sesame, rice, coconut and almond milk, fresh or store bought, unsweetened

ALL FRUITS: Except dates, which are acidic and high in sugar

VEGETABLE JUICES: Wheatgrass and other green juices, fresh or store bought. You can add some carrot juice or beet juice for taste. Keep your juices as green and full of chlorophyll as possible! Also, reconstituted green powders are excellent, and can be used throughout the day

ALKALINE PROTEINS: Almonds and almond butter, chestnuts, and Rice or hemp-based Protein Powders (Fermented soy products such as tempeh and tofu are alkaline, but since they can be challenging to digest, it is recommended that you limit your consumption of them while on this diet.)

ALKALINE SWEETENER: Stevia

ALKALIZING SPICES/SEASONINGS: Chili, cinnamon, curry, ginger, miso, mustard, sea salt, tamari

A LIVE FOOD, VEGAN DIET IS OPTIMAL FOR DETOXIFICATION! That's true, especially, because the meats and fish most of us have access to are toxic, due to the chemical, antibiotic and hormone exposures of the animals. However, how often have we put off making a change in our lives, or trying something new, out of the fear that if we can't do it "perfectly" (whatever that means!) we won't be successful. Please don't do that with this diet! That's the kind of thinking we want to transform. If you've picked up this book, you're ready to begin. Also, the "perfect diet" for one person, doesn't serve another. (*Eat Right 4 Your Blood Type*, by Dr. Peter D'Adamo, suggests our blood types may determine our optimal diet.) One of the goals of a detox diet is to clean your body out so that you feel so fantastic, you will crave foods that are good for you, without effort or a feeling of deprivation.

You may be saying, "I can't imagine living without sugar or my favorite glass of wine, even for three weeks." I have heard those very words from countless clients, who surprised themselves by not only doing it for three weeks, but much longer, because, simply, they were finally pain-free, food addiction-free, bloating-and-gas free and loving life.

Just remember: If you use animal protein on this detox diet, it must be organic!

And, one more thing ... no microwaves! Microwaves change the configuration of the molecules in our foods, and it takes our bodies an immense amount of energy to digest microwaved foods. Remember, this is all about making digestion as easy as possible...so, please, give yourself extra time and become friendly with your steamer, your oven (or convection oven), your double boiler, and your favorite non-Teflon skillet!

Your diet may consist of 30% of the following proteins, beans, nuts and grains. That means you may have one serving of an alkaline vegetable for every serving of proteins, beans, nuts and grains.

BEANS: Black beans, chick peas, kidney beans, lentils, pinto beans, red beans, soy beans, soy milk, white beans.

ORGANIC ANIMAL PROTEIN: As clean as possible

EGGS: Organic and preferably, locally grown!

NUTS: Cashews, peanuts and peanut butter, pecans, tahini, walnuts

GRAINS: Amaranth, quinoa, barley, rice, spelt, whole wheat, bran, millet, corn

SWEETENERS: Agave

The "NO DON'T EVEN THINK ABOUT IT" list:

Sugar, artificial sweeteners
Honey or maple syrup
White flour
Vinegar
Dairy
Processed or preserved foods
Fake fats (Use the fats on our "Good Fats" list only)
Coffee/alcohol/soda

SUGGESTED MEAL PLANS: The following meals are alkaline based and properly food combined. Because choosing alkaline foods – and identifying which they are – is new to most of us, it's helpful to have a map to go by!

BREAKFAST SUGGESTIONS:

Upon rising: The juice of one lemon in water,
Followed 10 minutes later by:
8 oz. of Fresh Green Vegetable Juice
Protein Smoothie with Rice,
Nut or Hemp Milk,
Banana or Frozen Berries and Protein Powder
Stir-fried Tofu with scrambled Bok Choy and Bean sprouts
Avocado Slivers on Sliced Green Apples or
*Julia's apple avocado Salad
Sliced Delicious Apples with Almond Butter
Almond Butter in *Baked Nutmeg Apples
 or *Poached Pears, or with fresh papaya
 (The following cereals and grains are slightly acidic, but can
 be comforting during a diet change!)

Hot Grain Cereal, such as rice, buckwheat groats or rye,
with rice milk
Oatmeal with rice milk
Spelt Toast with Butter

LUNCH SUGGESTIONS:

Salad Greens with *Julia's Fresh Lemon Dressing and
avocado slices
Grilled Red Peppers, Tofu and Mushrooms
Sprouted Greens with *Julia's Pumpkin Seed Sauce
*Summer Vegetable Soup
*Seaweed Salad Rolls
Spelt pasta and *Raw and spicy tomato sauce
Baked sweet potato with cinnamon and nutmeg,
and Garden Greens
Steamed or Grilled Vegetables and Basmati Rice

3 PM SNACK:

Fresh green juice or
PROTEIN SHAKE with Green Chlorophyll powder
and Banana

DINNER SUGGESTIONS:

Sprouted Greens and Chard with
*Guacamole, baked chips, & *Pine-nut Stuffed peppers
Steamed Artichoke with *Julia's Tahini Dressing,
Rice or Baked Potato, and Steamed or Grilled vegetables
Garden Salad with *Julia's Pumpkin Seed Dressing
Sweet potato and steamed or stir-fried Kale
Quinoa, corn on the cobb and salad
Spelt spaghetti with *Spicy Tomato Sauce
Pick-of-the-Garden Salad with Julia's Tahini Dressing

EVENING SNACK:

One piece of fresh fruit or
Spelt or Rice Cinnamon Toast
Sprouted wheat-free Live Manna Bread
*Julia's Guilt-free Oatmeal Cookies
(sweetened with Stevia or Agave)
*Baked Agave Apples or Nutmeg Baked Apples

RECIPES: Welcome To Julias Kitchen!

I've been adapting, creating and collecting recipes all my life. In the beginning, it was for survival – I had so few foods I could eat, I needed to learn ten things I could do with each one! And every recipe needed to be changed – and often still does. Luckily, early on, I fell in love with cooking and food preparation. The kitchen is the heart of my house, and with every meal, there's a big salad with home-made dressing. My kids have always loved vegetables, and eat raw red peppers as if they were crunchy apples. Here's a few of the recipes that my family and my clients have loved over the years. I made them as simple as possible to follow, because most of us are too busy to spend hours in the kitchen.

Recipes are made to be changed, so please change these, according to your taste and your own sensitivities.

Fresh Raw Almond Milk

2 cups raw organic almonds
1 tsp vanilla
1/8 tsp stevia or 1 tsp. agave (optional)

Soak the almonds overnight…and this milk is easiest to digest if the almonds are also sprouted, which removes the enzyme inhibitors. To sprout, drain the almonds and allow them to "grow" for 12-24 hours. Then blend with 5 cups filtered water, and strain in a very fine strainer or through cheesecloth. Refrigerate and enjoy! This is delicious over raw bananas or fresh berries, in smoothies, and as the base for a creamy salad dressing….nut milks have a multitude of uses! Excellent protein source for a transition diet…

Julia's Apple Avocado Salad

2 chopped apples
1 mashed avocado
2 tbsp. sesame or sunflower seeds, filberts or almonds
2 tbsp. raisins (optional)
juice of 1/2 lemon

pinch of nutmeg and cinnamon
1 tbps. apple juice concentrate (optional)

Mix together, chill and marinate 2-4 hours for best blend of flavors.
Delicious served in 1/2 a papaya with a squeeze of lime!
Serves 2.

Julia's Baked Nutmeg Apples

Scoop out the seeds of 2 apples;
Mix 1 tsp. butter or coconut oil, pinch of cinnamon
And 1/4 tsp of stevia and spread over apples
Cut in half two apples and scoop out the seeds
Place in pie plates and bake 45 min. at 350 degrees
Sprinkle with nutmeg before serving.
Serve warm or cold
Serves 2.

Julia's Agave Pears

Scoop the seeds out of two pears
Mix 1 tbsp. of agave, 1 tbps. Butter or coconut oil with
pinch of cinnamon and 1 tsp of   vanilla
Cut in half two pears and scoop out the seeds
Place pears in pie plates, and pour sauce over pears
Bake 30 min. at 350 degrees
Serve warm or cold
Serves 2.

Julia's Fresh Lemon Salad Dressing

This very simple dressing is a family favorite…and, no vinegar! Store
it in glass in the refrigerator

1/4 cup Fresh Lemon Juice
1/2 cup Olive Oil
1 tsp. Herbamare Seasoning or Herbal Seasoning of choice

Julia's Pumpkin Seed Sauce

I discovered nut sauces when I was at Hippocrates Health Institute, where they serve them as delicious, raw protein substitutes. You can experiment with your own versions of the recipe below.

1/2 cup beet juice
1 cup carrot juice
1 cup soaked pumpkin seeds (or sunflower seeds)
1/2 tbsp. lemon juice
1/3 cup olive or avocado oil
Add to taste: 1 clove garlic, 1/4 tsp dill, parlsey and pinch of cayenne, 1/2 cup sliced scallions, cilantro, 1 tsp. Himalayan pink sea salt

Blend till creamy, adding the olive oil as needed;
and chill before serving

Nut dressings are even healthier for us when they are sprouted. To do that, soak one cup of seeds or nuts overnight in water. In the morning, drain the water and allow the seeds to sprout for 24 hours. They are then ready for using in sauces or milks, and can be refrigerated as well, for 2-3 days.

Summer Vegetable Soup

In the summer, our soup is full of fresh vegetables from the local farmer's market. You'll notice there aren't any tomatoes in this soup, and that's because cooked tomatoes are very acidic. This soup is very alkalizing, perfect for cleansing and healing diets. The vegetables can be varied, depending on what you find organic at the vegetable stand or grocery store.

4 chopped zucchini
2 chopped sweet potatoes or golden potatoes
1 stalk of celery, chopped
6 green or yellow summer squashes, chopped
1 chopped red onion
3 ears corn, grated off the cob

1 clove garlic
1 cup fresh snap peas
1 cup fresh green beans, chopped
1 tsp. Himalayan pink sea salt
1 tsp. pepper or cayenne to taste
Optional: 1/4 a chopped beet

Put all ingredients in large soup pot and add 2-4 quarts of water, or until the water comes 3 inches over the top of the ingredients.

Cover and bring to a boil, then simmer for 30-45 min, until the potatoes are cooked.

Serves 4.

In the winter, we make this soup with kale, yams and leeks, and whatever surprises us at our local farmer's market. Sometimes we're in a hurry, and add frozen organic corn and peas. And I love creamed soups, so I often take a few cups of this soup and toss it into the blender for a soothing, late night snack.

Seaweed Salad Rolls

If you haven't experimented with seaweeds, you're missing a phenomenal taste treat that's loaded with vitamins, minerals and natural iodine. These rolls are excellent by themselves, on top of greens, rice or served as an appetizer to your entrée of choice.

One package of dulse
One package of arame
One chopped red onion
One chopped or diced red pepper
One large chopped tomato
1/4 cup olive oil
1/4 cup lemon juice
1 tsp. garlic powder
pinch of cayenne pepper, to taste
2 tsp grated fresh ginger
One chopped avocado
Nori (a dried flat seaweed used for sushi)

Soak the arame 30-45 minutes, till soft. It will still be a
bit crunchy. Strain and pour in large mixing bowl.
Rinse the dulse and soak for five minutes; strain and
pour in large mixing bowl.
Add the seaweed to all the other ingredients, except the Nori.
Lay the Nori flat on a table or board, and add 2-3 tbsp.
of the seaweed salad per Nori strip, and roll.
Keeps three days in the refrigerator.
Serves 4.

Spelt pasta with Raw and Spicy Tomato Sauce

Tomatos become very acidic cooked, but they make a
wonderful raw sauce over greens or pasta. There are
many variations to wheat pasta that are delicious and
gluten-free. Our favorites are rice and spelt.

1 Package spelt or rice pasta
6 large tomatoes
2 cloves Garlic
pinch cayenne
Optional: 1 chopped onion (raw, carmelized or grilled), 1 cup finely
chopped leeks or scallions, 1 bunch finely chopped cilantro and/or
fresh basil
1/4 cup olive oil
1 tsp. Himalayan pink sea salt
Chop tomatoes into cubes and add all other ingredients.
Pour over warm pasta
Serves 4.

Julia's Tangy Guacamole

2 avocados, chopped and smashed till smooth
the juice of 1-2 lemons
1 tsp Himalayan pink sea salt, pinch cayenne or 1 tsp.
Herbamare seasoning
Optional: 1/2 chopped onion, chopped scallions or
chopped fresh cilantro, or 1 clove fresh garlic
Mix all ingredients, chill and serve
Serves 2.

Pinenut Stuffed Red Peppers

Red peppers are a huge favorite at my house; we use them for everything! They have more vitamin C than most fruits, and are a perfect partner to the rich, savory flavor of pinenuts.

Two red peppers, with seeds removed
1 cup pinenuts
1 cup chopped celery
1/4 cup chopped scallions
1 clove garlic
1/2 cup olive oil, or as needed
2 cups fresh basil leaves
Fresh cilantro or dill (optional)
dash cayenne

Combine all ingredients except the peppers In a food processor; or use a mortar and pestle, and add the vegetables after the pinenuts have been well blended to a thick paste
Stuff peppers with the pinenut mixture and serve
Serves 2.

Julia's Tahini Dressing

1 cup raw tahini
1 cup lemon juice
2 cloves garlic
1 tsp agave (optional)
1 tsp pink Himalayan Sea Salt
dash cayenne

Blend and chill....serve over greens

Guilt-free Oatmeal Cookies

1 cup oat or oatmeal flour, preferably from steelcut oats
1 cup spelt flour
8 tbs. butter, melted

1/4 cup agave or 2 tsp. white stevia powder
1 egg
1 tsp vanilla
1 tsp salt
1 tsp baking powder

Preheat oven to 350 degrees

Mix all ingredients in a large bowl with spoon or
mixer; Drop onto cookie sheet and bake…
10-14 minutes, until golden

Sugar-free Cinnamon Toast

1/4 tsp. white powder stevia
1 tsp. cinnamon
2 pieces spelt or rice bread, toasted
1 tsp. butter

Mix the stevia with the cinnamon.
Butter the toast hot, and sprinkle on the
mixture … enjoy!

DURING YOUR DETOX DIET:

Drink lemon water throughout the day!

And Consider the following:

Supplements:

Food enzymes with each meal

Probiotic, once a day without food

Lymph Cleansing.

10 minutes a day on rebounder or trampoline

Dry skin brushing.

Colon Cleansing:

Colon cleansing product for removing plaque from the colon

If you have IBS, colitis or a sensitive colon, two herbs that are commonly found in colon cleansing products — Senna and Cascara Sagrada – may cause irritation, gas or bloating. Try Aloe Vera juice instead! 1 – 4 tbs. 2 x a day

The above 21-day detox is designed to help your body flush toxins, and can assist anyone dealing with fatigue, Candida, constipation, metabolism issues, as well as degenerative diseases that are associated with acidity and toxicity. We suggest our active clients consume at least 50-75 grams of protein a day, but we have seen that most detox diets don't include enough protein to sustain busy people!

On the Detox Diet, you may choose to reduce the amount of animal protein you are used to consuming. Please supplement that with nut milks, nut sauces or rice or hemp-based protein powders, which usually have 10 to 15 grams of protein per serving. They are an excellent, easy-to-digest way to make that up extra protein that we all need.

The following case history is a great example of how one of our clients turned his life around by going on the 21-day detox diet.

ALEX

Alex, a young man in his late thirties, was a former football player in college. He owned and managed a nightclub in town, which-meant late nights, late meals and lots of alcohol. Even though he looked healthy and strong with no apparent physical problems, his handsome baby face was bloated and red, he was 35 pounds over-weight and not a bit happy about it. When he spoke to me, he said his goal was to lose weight, regain his energy and clean out his liver. Apparently, his business partner had done our cleanse the year before, had lost 40 pounds, and was beating him at basketball and everything else. (Competition can be a terrific motivator).

"Game on!" Alex called out to me, as I outlined my cleansing program for him, but I had my doubts about how strictly he'd adhere to my suggestions. Fresh, organic foods, juices and green smoothies were a whole new world for him since his only previous experience with blenders had been making margaritas! But like so many of my clients, as we got to know each other, he told me he was suffering from a lot more than constipation, gas, weight gain and low energy. He'd been recently diagnosed with ulcers, and gout ran in his family.

"My wife is pregnant and I don't want to be a beached whale of a dad!" he said. "The doctors gave me meds for my ulcers, but I read up on them, and there's a whole hell of a lot of side effects."

I had a proposal for him. "This detox and diet program is a drastically different lifestyle than the one you have," I said. "Can you commit to this 100% for 21 days, and give it a shot?"

"I already have!" he said. And he did.

In 21 days, Alex lost 15 pounds, and who knows how much gas. We wish we could have measured. When he spoke about the fire in his belly, it wasn't gas any more. Rather, he was referring to his passion for his new hobby: Cooking! His plan was to continue with the program until he lost 20 more pounds, and then see what it would take to maintain, which is the most challenging part of any lifestyle change, let alone for someone running a nightclub.

I saw Alex last week, and he was excited to show off, as he calls it, "my all new-Six pack – but not the kind in cans my gut used to be filled with!"

When I asked him what he was filling his gut with these days, he said, "I don't always food combine perfectly but I always take my food enzymes! They're lifesavers if I eat late. And I still drink occasionally, but that day to day chugging is out. Especially anything with sugar! If I feel any grumbling going on down south, I get radical for a few days and all's good."

"What do you mean by 'radical?'" I wanted to know.

"No junk," he said, "no flour, no cheese, no sugar, no alcohol. I take a wheatgrass shot in the afternoon and I test my pH. Those green smoothies are my breakfast norm – who woulda' thought?! I've discovered that tri-tip steak just kills me, damn! But it's worth it not to be doubled up after a bar-b-que, so it's salmon on the grill these days. With salad and no sour cream dips, either. But hey, my stomach pain is gone. I went off the meds last month. I can live without sour cream!"

He went on, "I splurged on my birthday and had chocolate cake. I told myself I'd give the rest of the cake to my brother to take home, but at the last minute, I just tucked it into the back of the freezer and the next day I had a little piece, and the next. By the end of that week, my stomach was killing me. I had so much gas, I looked more pregnant than my wife! You told me white flour and sugar can really upset the stomach, but I had to learn the hard way."

Everyone's maintenance regime is different, but until we're feeling flat-out fabulous for a week straight and then a month straight and then three months straight, we aren't in a very good position to know what to keep and what to throw out.

Alex went back on his program for two weeks to straighten himself out. And it worked. "Babies take more energy than I ever imagined," he said, "so its lucky this papa is up for it. On my day off, I put my new daughter in the stroller and we cruise the farmer's market. And there's stuff I won't buy at the grocery store so I'm not up looking at it in the middle of the night or when I get home from work. That really helps. Now, I eat before I go to the club, and I drink lemon water all night. Sometimes I even have lemon in my club soda.'"

Alex winked at me, because he knew I wasn't a fan of carbonation. But from daily vodka sours and fried chicken wings to club soda and lemon – that's a win!!

PART THREE:

Dos And Don'ts Of Detox

CHAPTER ELEVEN:
Acid/Alkaline Balance

After years of research and experimentation, I have learned that stress and our emotions have more to do with our health than anything else. But make no mistake. I'm not implying that your food allergies are "all in your head," though the doctors told me that over and over as a kid. But, do you know what? In a certain sense, they were right, in that my head had a lot to do with my ill health – but not the way they thought.

A person cannot simply "will" physical symptoms away or pretend they don't exist. While the stress of my emotional environment and my internal stew created a very acid system, which in turn created allergies, the allergies and reactions were very real. The acid was real. It had to be recognized and dealt with along with the emotional patterns that were the source of these difficult symptoms.

Just as my physical symptoms were real, so are yours. There, I've said it – you're not crazy. Your physical pain and discomfort are creating a lot of stress and negativity because *negativity is acidity*. This leads us to studying our pH as a whole new way to drop acid!

Scientifically speaking, pH is the measurement of the degree of saturation of the hydrogen ion in a substance or solution. That means that your pH tells the tale of whether your body tends to be alkaline or acidic. It's so easy, you can lick or pee on a pH strip right now and you'll know in two seconds how balanced you are. 6.4 to 7.4 is the range we want to be in. Where are you? It is important to know because an imbalance in the body's pH may lead to:

- Low energy
- Slow digestion and elimination
- Hormone concerns
- Depression
- Cramps
- Headaches
- Weight gain
- Joint discomfort.

More serious symptoms are:

- Cardiovascular weakness
- Bladder and kidney disease
- Immune breakdown
- Stressed liver function
- Yeast/Candida overgrowth
- Pancreatic dysfunction

You've heard me mention the acid/alkaline balance that is necessary for health, but do you know what that means? The extensive science that backs this approach was pioneered by biologist Dr. Robert Young. He says that the body is alkaline by nature. Acid comes in as the body goes about its business of breathing, moving, digesting. In other words, the body must maintain alkalinity at all times, and yet every function the body does, by necessity, creates acids.

Gastric acids such as hydrochloric acid in the stomach combine with foods and liquids and initiate chemical reactions that break down nutrients so they can be digested. Acids are key elements in powering the body! They start up hundreds of organic and chemical processes so we call them the "starters" of life. They are not bad for us and we can't live without them! But they get out of balance because of our lifestyles.

Electrolyte minerals which have the capacity to conduct electricity and are literally the energy of life, buffer the acids that these functions create, and maintain a perfect acid/alkaline balance. They allow the twenty-two-plus enzymes the body needs to digest food to exist and work properly. Without this balance, we are on our way to malnutrition (which leads to disease and addiction) because we are not absorbing any nutrients. Rather, we are literally starving! And, without this delicate balance, our bowels, which are alkaline by nature in contrary to the rest of our internal organs, become acidic. To protect itself, the intestines make a thick mucous barrier inside the colon to guard itself from this acid bath. It is this barrier that we called mucoid plaque.

At this point, if the body doesn't maintain an alkaline balance, the cells begin to die. To keep that from happening when there aren't enough electrolytes to buffer digestive acids, the body goes to other parts of itself to find the electrolytes it needs. It will do anything it takes to keep the pH balanced, just like it will do anything to keep the temperature balanced. So, it will literally cannibalize itself to survive, using our electrolyte buffers from our cells to re-balance us. As a result, our bodies run out of these buffers very quickly because most of us are on very acidic diets.

For instance, if the body is constantly using the calcium we already have to neutralize the acids we consume, we're prone to osteoporosis. When we over-eat acid foods, our healthy red blood cells turn into bacteria and yeast! This is the foundation of degenerative disease.

In his book, *Cleanse and Purify Thyself,* Dr. Rich Anderson tells us that when the digestive system goes from alkaline to acid, the following problems occur:

- Gallstones form.
- Hydrochloric acid, imperative for digestion, is impaired.
- Acids enter the intestines and mucoid plaque develops.
- Sugars can't be broken down into a usable form, causing blood sugar issues.
- Mucus, cholesterol and lymph congestion decrease circulation, leading to poor memory and foggy thinking, among other things.
- Cells and organs starve.
- Free radicals escalate.
- Immune function weakens
- Disease develops.

When we eat alkaline-forming foods, we have more than enough electrolytes to buffer any acids are in the foods. When we eat acid foods or have stress (which most of us do), there are not enough electrolytes to buffer the acids. What is left is an excess of acids and the depletion of electrolytes. Where electrolytes are used by the body to buffer acids, the tissue or organ involved is compromised. Circulation is also compromised, and where we have poor circulation, acids accumulate. At a certain point of deterioration, cancer can develop.

One of the first place electrolytes are compromised is in the stomach. Dr. Bernard Jenson, a renowned doctor and educator, taught us that over eighty percent of the people who go to a hospital have no hydrochloric acid production. That's why HCL, or hydrochloric acid, is often recommended to our clients. Without it, we may digest and absorb very little of what we eat. And, if we have too much HCL, we get ulcers. Both conditions can be effected greatly by proper acid/alkaline balance.

Raymond Francis, an internationally recognized leader in the emerging field of optimal health maintenance says in his book, *Never Be Sick Again*, that if all our cells are healthy, our body will be resilient. His theory is that disease is caused by one of two things:

- Deficiency – the cell is not getting what it must have.
  or
- Toxicity – the cell is being poisoned by something that alters or stops its function.

Dr. Young, in his analysis of live blood, has seen that emotions can have twice the effect on our blood as food can! That is so important, because it's easy to assume that a "perfect diet" alone will make us feel great and, vice versa, it's easy to assume that if we fall off the wagon with our diets, we'll get sick. Not necessarily! A lot of that depends on what we're feeling at the time, how aware we allow ourselves to become of those feelings, and how we choose to act on what those feelings are trying to tell us!

When we are acidic, the way to alkalize our body is to ingest at least 70% alkaline foods until our pH strips measure 6.4. When that pH strip is measuring 6.4, it's a glorious day! Remember Joanne, whom you met at the beginning of this book? I wish I had captured Joanne on video one month after we met, as she came running into my office holding her test strip in her hand, showing a brilliant 6.4. She was shouting, "I DID IT! I DID IT!" all the way down the hall!

119

If you noticed that we've been talking a lot about being too acidic, do you wonder if that's the only thing we need to worry about? Can we become too alkaline? YES! Though it's more uncommon, it happens. Over-alkalinity creates serious congestion in the body and a deterioration of the vital organs. It can occur from using over-alkaline water and not testing one's pH. We've had clients buy alkaline water systems and watch their health go down the tubes! They weren't conscious of testing themselves, thinking there was no down-side to alkalinity, only to acidity. Testing our pH can save us from killing ourselves with our good intentions!

ALKALINE WATER

Alkaline water is a water system designed to allow our bodies to flush acid. There are many companies that make them, but the one we have in our Clinic is from Kangen. Because you can adjust the machine to boost the alkalinity in the water it creates, you can easily boost your alkalinity, should your morning pH strip show you are acidic.

Alkaline water has been used in over 100 hospitals and medical clinics in Japan for over 30 years to treat a number of disease conditions. International scientific studies have shown the benefits of "restructured through ionization" hexagonal water. This ionization process alters the structure of the water, making it more bio-available to your body, and increasing nutrient absorption at the cellular level.

Because water makes up 70% of the body's weight, what could be more important than the type of water you drink? Here are some of the positive benefits from alkaline water:

- Improves oxygenation to the cells
- Removes waste from the cells

- Lubricates the joints
- Regulates body temperature
- Improves respiratory function
- Increases athletic performance

My Kangen water machine has five settings:

- 1.5: This setting is great for removing oil based pesticides from produce, kitchen grease and grime, as a detergent to unclog drains for an effective, healthy chemical-free cleaning for homes, as a poultice for hot, inflamed areas, and as a spray on sun burns.
- 8.5-9: This setting is for cooking and drinking as it contains large quantities of negatively charged ions which act as antioxidants.
- Clean water, 7.0 (neutral): This setting makes chlorine-free water and removes impurities while keeping the buffering minerals we need, such as calcium, magnesium, and sodium potassium. (Reverse osmosis water removes this.)
- Acid water/Beauty water, 5.5 (not for drinking): Beauty water has astringent properties that are good for the skin and scalp. It firms the pores like a toner and works well for other skin problems like psoriasis, rashes, eczema and acne.
- Strong acidic water, 2.4 (not for drinking): This is a disinfectant for germs. It kills viruses, staph, MRSA, strep, fungus and Ecoli in 30 seconds to one minute. Use this water setting as first aid for cuts and scrapes.

CHAPTER TWELVE:
Making It Easy

An ideal formula for balance is 70% alkaline and 30% acid. But how do we know we're eating an exactly 70/30 diet? Are we going around measuring the pH of everything we eat? That would make us crazy, and that causes acidity! Here are some tools we give our clients to make going alkaline a lot easier than passing your sixth grade science final.

FREEZE DRIED GREENS OR LIQUID CHLOROPHYLL

About thirty years ago, when I first started testing my urine and learning about pH, there were not dozens of choices of freeze-dried, mineral-rich green powders and liquid chlorophylls available to make going alkaline easier. So I was juicing greens all day. Although nothing takes the place of fresh juice, especially if you're seriously ill, my job is giving my clients tools that are practical as well as effective. Freeze-dried powdered greens are one of my favorites.

Start with one teaspoon a day in water. This can be increased to a tablespoon twice a day as your body becomes used to it. Drink in water, add it to your smoothies in the morning, or use it as a pick-me-up in the afternoon. Though these greens are not toxic in larger

123

amounts, ingesting may cause detox symptoms such as loose bowels or headaches while your body is getting used to it.

LEMONS

Drinking the juice of a squeezed lemon in water is the most alkalizing thing we can do for ourselves. Start the day with a warm cup of lemon water (if you wish, sweeten with stevia, a natural and alkalizing sweetener) Although it may seem that citrus foods are acidic, they actually have an alkalizing effect on the body. Having a pitcher of water with lemons next to you during the day is a great way to drink more water, while you are also cleansing your liver, kidneys and gall bladder.

USE FOOD ENZYMES (described in detail later)
ADD CALCIUM AND MAGNESIUM
TAKE EXTRA VITAMIN D3
GET PLENTY OF OMEGA 3'S

ADD PROBIOTICS

Probiotics are the friendly bacteria that support a normal colon and the prevention of yeasts, Candida, bacteria and parasites. Taking a daily probiotic increases not only colon function and promotes regular elimination, but also strengthens the immune system and helps regulate hormone balance. Look for a dairy free probiotic. This will need to be kept in the refrigerator.

DRINK PLENTY OF WATER

I once attended a lecture by Dr. Brian Clement, head of Hippocrates Health Institute, who said that dehydration is one of the top five conditions that are most detrimental to our health! When my clients, or my kids, complain of a headache, or are feeling cranky, the first thing I'll ask is, "How much water have you had today?" Signs of dehydration are the following: Acid reflux, Allergies, Asthma, Constipation, Cramps, Depression, Headaches, pH imbalance, and weight gain.

According to Dr. Philip Golgia, author of *Turn up The Heat, Unlock the Fat-burning Power of Your Metabolism*, the correct amount of daily water we need is one ounce per pound of body weight. Some people feel better if they don't drink with meals, so drink water in between. Squeezing a lemon in the water not only alkalinizes it, but may make it more appealing if you're not in the habit of drinking water. Since water, the cheapest medicine we've got, is the vehicle that moves the toxins out of the lymph, we may as well use it.

CLEAN THE COLON
EAT A 70/30 ALKALINE/ACID FOODS DIET

After you start the 21-day Detox, if you notice your body is acidic, add an extra green drink during the day, and add lemon to your water. If your body does not get anywhere near alkaline during the 21-day program, you may be dealing with a serious health issue and should see your medical practitioner. Medications, stress, and dehydration all affect our acid/alkaline balance.

When I started healing my body, I was dealing with serious health issues, and it took six months for me to become alkaline. A doctor friend of mine said he reminds his "patients" that the word has a meaning: PATIENCE. It will take some patience and fortitude to say good-bye for 21 days to:

- Sugar and artificial sugar substitutes
- Alcohol
- Coffee
- Soda
- White Flour
- White Vinegar
- Preserved and Processed Foods
- Fried Foods
- Fake Fats such as Margarine
- Dairy

Sugar is the most acidifying substance a person can ingest. I don't even call it a food because it has no food value. One tablespoon of refined sugar can lower the immune system by up to fifty percent for four hours. It feeds food and substance addictions and is one of the biggest contributors to depression, heart disease, cancer and diabetes. Sugar, along with antibiotics create acidity and feed CANDIDA, a natural yeast bacteria that grows in our colon. If you have any of the following symptoms, you may have a Candida overgrowth: Bladder or yeast infections, gas, bloating, brain fog, fatigue, depression, anxiety, mood swings, trouble concentrating, headaches, constipation, allergies and PMS.

I've seen among my clients that a sugar-free diet has radically improved their ability to stay alkaline, to be pro-active with a clean diet, and to support their desire to steer clear of drugs and alcohol. I usually recommend my clients maintain this diet for at least three months, along with an herbal supplement and a probiotic to combat Candida, which is very common, but not always diagnosed by doctors. If you feel you have it, check with a health practitioner who is experienced in diagnosing and treating Candida naturally. Diet alone is not always enough to completely eliminate Candida; an experienced practitioner may recommend protocols that include herbs such as pau d'arco" and grapefruit seed extract.

It sounds so dramatic to say that sugar is poison, so we'll say only that for some of us, it really is. The only way to find out how it affects you is to go without it for 21 days. Then, as you add some back in your diet, really pay attention to how you feel. Ask yourself the hard questions, like I would if you were in my office! And don't forget, artificial sweeteners create acidity and have been proven to be cancerforming. That is why I recommend Stevia and agave as safe, natural sweeteners.

Ask yourself, How do you feel after you eat sugar? Do you have mood swings, loss of concentration, sadness or anger? How do you feel the day after consuming sugar? Have you noticed a correlation between your sugar intake and your tendency to catch a cold or the flu? If you are strong and healthy, with no blood sugar issues like hypoglycemia or diabetes, your body will probably be able to tolerate some sugar in your life. But moderation is always the key. Look at these statistics:

- In 1850, the average American was consuming 12 pounds of sugar a year
- Today, in 2011, that number is up to 160 pounds.

And that difference is what's doing us in.

ALCOHOL/COFFEE/SODA

Do I really need to explain why you shouldn't drink these things while you're on a cleanse? What I do want to say, however, is that coffee has only one decent use during a cleanse: for colonics. We consider this a much better place to put coffee than in your mouth.

WHITE FLOUR

White flour has very little food value. Kids would be much better off eating a healthy, wholegrain cereal with rice milk and a banana than the sugary cereals we see on TV, and that many of us grew up with. Because white flour is so acidic, removing it from the diet for 21 days gives our digestive systems a chance to breathe, literally.

Our goal is to eat a diet as close to our ancestors as possible, because that's what makes our bodies happy and healthy. If our ancestors had eaten 200 pounds of white flour a year like most Americans do, I might not be writing this book because we might not be here!

Have you ever made glue for an art project with water and white flour? It works amazingly! OK, now picture your intestines with inches of that glue stuck inside it – *for years!* It's not pretty. And it's not white anymore. The worst part is that fewer and fewer nutrients are able to get through that glue (called mucoid plaque) and make it into your bloodstream. At the same tine, less and less waste is able to get out. This causes constipation or diarrhea or both.

WHITE VINEGAR

This is extremely acidic, so I suggest you replace it with raw apple cider vinegar. But if you struggle with yeast infections or bladder infections, you may be better off without even apple cider vinegar. Use lemon on your salads instead.

PRESERVATIVES/PROCESSED FOODS

It's time to clean out your refrigerator and your pantry. But don't plan fifteen minutes for this activity. Set aside from two to four hours and consider it a huge gift to yourself. If you end up disposing of $200 worth of processed foods, it will easily be a hundred times less than what you would pay your doctor for the ailments these dangerous substances cause! Sorry for beating a dead horse or rather flogging a swollen liver, but once again, I want to remind you that these "non-foods" are loaded with chemicals that we do not poop or pee out. We don't sweat them out either. They stay in our bodies until we consciously, deliberately, and often painfully detox them. If we don't, they will eventually make us very sick.

We begin by storing them in our lymph, our colon and our liver. Then they make their way into our breasts, our reproductive systems, our brains and our nervous systems, which is why these chemicals not only make us sick, but also make us crazy. I don't know about you, but in my life, I attempt to accomplish about twenty things a day, including, where the heck did I put that piece of paper Luke needs signed for his baseball coach? I can't afford chemicals scrambling the precious brain cells that survived my youth!

I must add here that though I'm a believer in birth control, I'd rather it not be in the form of hormones my kids eat in their foods. Have you stopped to notice the three-page novella of side effects written in tiny letters on the back of a pill bottle? It might read something like: "Can cause suicide, homicide, diarrhea, chance of strokes, psychotic episodes, exploding tendons, ruptured muscles, etc." Nothing like that is attached to the processed chicken tenders, but it ought to be.

If there is one message I want to get across in this book, it's that our great-great-to-the-millionth-power grandmother did not drink a Diet Coke while she was writing her to-do list on the cave wall. Moses may never have gotten that gang across the desert alive in 40 days if they'd been eating French fries and drinking soda. (Sugar is extremely dehydrating!)

Well, even today, your body still doesn't recognize sugar and chemicals as food. These substances instantly create acid, which causes pain in your gut and a lot of gas. If you're trying to lose weight or speed up your metabolism, eating processed foods and chemical additives is like shoveling sand at the beach during a windstorm. It just won't go where you want it to go. So, head over to your pantry and fridge and read the labels on the foods. If you see preservatives and additives on a label, toss it. Please don't say to yourself, "I just won't eat this stuff for 21 days!" If it's in front of you, you'll probably eat it, so why sabotage yourself? It takes enough willpower to control yourself when you're out. Your home should be a stress-free zone when it comes to diet temptations. And then, why would you ever want to go back to processed food after 21 days of cleansing?

If you are the only person in your family doing this cleanse, you'll have far more success if you enlist everyone's support up front, even if you can't talk them into joining you. If you don't get their support, I have a lot of compassion for you, because I've worked with many clients in that situation, and Wes and I have been there ourselves. It's much tougher, but you can do it anyway! The truth is that food is one of the most emotional subjects and it's complicated.

Whatever your partner's reaction is to your decision to cleanse your body, here's one of my favorite laws from Miguel Ruiz's wonder ful book, *THE FOUR AGREEMENTS*: *It's not about you. It's not personal to you.*

It often feels threatening to partners and families when we change our habits, because they are afraid of being left behind, whether they say it out loud or not. They may be afraid that they themselves can't change, even if they want to. And they may interpret your desire to change, even doing a temporary cleanse, as a message that the life you are living with them is unsatisfactory. Then they escalate this imagined dissatisfaction in their minds from 1 to 100. So when you discuss what you are doing with family or friends, stay with your feelings, because no one can argue with feelings. Explanations and pleading are useless. Just say what you need in the simplest terms, and tell them how it makes you feel to be supported or not supported. You'll discover that when you come from your heart and not from your head, you'll be much harder to argue with.

One last tip: You might also mention to your mate that if your tummy wasn't hurting, if your gut wasn't bloated, and if you had any energy at all, you would feel a lot more hot and horny. That one works every time and guess what? It's true!!

FRIED FOODS/ FAKE OILS

OK, let's blow up the myth of the benefits of the non-fat or low-fat diet. *We need fats* to think, to have energy, to reproduce. Without them, we starve. But while the right kinds of fats help our cells regulate the passage of materials, artificial oils and fried fats make us fat and sick. This is because eating the wrong kinds of fats causes our cells to malfunction, resulting in just about any disease you are susceptible to. (We all have our Achilles heels, and yes, genetics do matter.)

What are essential fatty acids? We've all heard the term, which refers to fats that the body needs and can't make. Their specific shape is critical to the way they work in forming a cell membrane, making them the perfect brick-and-mortar to build cell walls. When oils are heated over 329 degrees, as most supermarket oils are, they become toxic and are called "trans fats." They become leaky and brittle, and when we have lots leaky and brittle cells in our body, then, Houston, we have a problem!

Considering the above information, I suggest you throw out everything in your pantry or fridge that is not high quality olive oil, organic cold-pressed nut oils like flaxseed and hemp oil, organic butter, ghee and essential fatty acid supplements. Wave good-bye to vegetable shortening and oils from the supermarket that are not marked "raw and organic."

Make sure you use at least 2 tbsp. of cold-pressed, organic oil daily, maybe in your smoothie, in your salad or sprinkle on top of your vegetables. This is absolutely essential to high energy. And do yourself a big favor after your 21-day cleanse: never use margarine again.

DAIRY PRODUCTS

Contrary to popular ads, milk does *not* do a body good. It was designed for calves, not humans, and even mother cows don't nurse their babies with pasteurized milk. If they did, their calves would die of starvation. Did you know that 70% of the world's population do not drink milk? According to the book, "*Eat 4 Your Blood Type*", many ethnic groups are largely lactose intolerant, including Asians, Africans,

Latinos, Indians, Greeks, Arabs and Eskimos. This is because their ancestors never drank cow milk or ate cheese.

We've found this research to be true in our practice. Actually, we have found that most our clients do better without dairy in their diets. The exception seems to be our friends from France and the Scandinavian countries, who have been eating dairy for centuries. But for most of us, the phosphorous in cow's milk actually inhibits calcium from being absorbed, which is pretty ironic for those who drink milk for the sole purpose of getting calcium.

A note about milk: If and when you add it back into your diet, the minute you feel a cold or flu coming on, until you're well again, out it goes! Dairy products coat the intestines with mucus, and as you clean out your diet, you might notice they do the same to your sinuses and lungs. Guess what they make Elmer's glue with? Milk.

When it comes to butter, you may be surprised to find out that it is not really a dairy product. It's a fat. Most people allergic to dairy can digest butter, and we recommend it over margarine. If you use ghee, which is clarified butter, there is absolutely no dairy in it at all, and it is very alkalizing.

For kids, dairy products along with sugar are often the cause of allergies, ear infections and asthma. Neither of my kids have ever had an ear infection, a blessing I attribute that to the fact that I nursed them until they were 3 and I kept them off wheat, dairy and sugar for their first 8 years. Yes, really, 8 years. Now that they have turned into incredibly healthy teenagers who rarely miss school, I can say that bringing rice milk ice cream to those kindergarten birthday parties was worth it! I guess its time to own up to lying to Luke and Hana by telling them for years that carob was chocolate!

CHAPTER THIRTEEN:
Food Combining

If losing weight and speeding up your metabolism is a priority for you, then food combining may be your secret weapon. Food combining was originally popularized in the book, *Fit For Life*, an excellent read by Harvey and Marilyn Diamond. Thousands of people have lost weight on *Fit for Life*. But, for me, it all started in Beverly Hills!

Do you remember a book called, *The Beverly Hills Diet*, written in the 80's by Judy Mazel? I read it when I was 22, and I don't think I'd digested any of my food in 22 years – before I experimented with what she had to say about food combining. This book offered me an understanding of digestive enzymes, and the fact that our bodies can only digest certain food groups at a time. I know the words "it changed my life" sound so cliché, but it changed my life!!

Food combining is based on chemistry. To digest carbohydrates, we need the enzyme *amylase*, which is made in our saliva so we can pre-digest food in our mouth. For the digestion of protein, we need hydrochloric acid which is made in our stomach. The saliva in our mouth thins when we eat protein in order to get it into our stomachs efficiently. But if we eat these two foods, carbohydrates and proteins together – as in the classic American sandwich, which has turkey and bread, or eggs and toast, or pasta and meat sauce – we have a digestive mess.

Let's say you're having a turkey burger for lunch – trying to be healthy. You're chewing each bite slowly, the way you were taught, and the food is making its way down to your stomach. The turkey is mashed in with the carbohydrates and the stomach acids are working away, trying to find it!

Ok, now the food is lying in your stomach for hours, as your stomach acids are working on the protein, and the carbohydrate – the bread – starts to ferment. This is when the heartburn, belching and gas starts! In the small intestine, the enzymes for carbohydrates have to work harder because the *amylase* in your mouth didn't have much time to do its job. Meanwhile, the protein begins to rot and the bread is already putrefying. This leads to constipation, stomach aches, indigestion, acid reflux, and allergies. Why allergies? Because the undigested food may pass through the bowel skin into the blood and lymph. It's not food anymore. It's a toxic substance that the body doesn't recognize and can't use or flush out.

I used the example of a turkey sandwich here because of a personal experience. I was six months pregnant with my first child, Luke, and was finishing up a few hours of errands with a stop at the market to get something for dinner. I was starved! I hadn't planned very well and hadn't eaten all day. At this point, food combining had been a part of my life for over a decade but I figured, what the heck! A little voice in my head said, "Julia, for God's sakes, what's the big deal?" So I ordered a fresh turkey sandwich and ate it.

Within two hours I was doubled over with cramps, certain I was having a miscarriage. I had had three already, I was completely freaked out, and it never occurred to me that this much pain could be caused by gas. But people go to the emergency room all the time with gas pains like I was having! Sure enough, after I lay in the fetal position for what seemed like forever, I went to the bathroom and passed enough gas to light about 18 matches! And then my stomach was calm and baby safe!

Food combining was developed in the US by Dr. Howard Hay in the 1930's, although it's really much older, having been based on how humans ate as we evolved. Ten thousand years ago, we became farmers, but before that, for 990,000 years – 99% of our evolution – we were hunter/gatherers. In the morning, perhaps our Great-to the millionth power Aunt Edna picked berries and that was breakfast for the tribe. For dinner, Great-to-the-millionth-power Uncle Ezra killed a bison and that was all that was served for dinner. There were not twelve things on the dinner table.

It was in the last one percent of our evolution when mixed food became available by farming, ranching, and the storing of supplies. Mixing foods seems "normal" to us, but biogenetically, we were created for healthy food combining!

And yet, there is one group of humans who still have their gut instincts: Kids! Instead of being called "biogenetically brilliant," they're usually called "picky eaters." Although both my kids loved a variety of foods from the time they were little, they wanted everything separate and plain. God forbid we would put the banana on the cereal. It would not get eaten!

Here is food combining made simple:

- Eat proteins with vegetables and fats.

- Eat carbohydrates with vegetables and fats.

- Eat fruits alone

I had a food combining chart pinned on my refrigerator when I started, to make it easier, so the food combining chart at the end of the chapter is for you. I am aware that this way of eating, like so many things I am writing about, is controversial. But for me, the proof is in doing something and reaping results. After struggling with painful digestion, bleeding ulcers, gas, the constipation/diarhhea cycle, diverticulitis and colitis, I was willing to try anything. Because my hypoglycemia was so bad – that's low blood sugar (my dad was a diabetic) – not only did my stomach hurt after every meal, my blood sugar also plummeted. It got to the point where I hated eating because an hour after a meal, I would have no energy. That was until I tried food combining and everything changed for the better. Oh, and one other miracle that I'm about to discuss in the next chapter: DIGESTIVE ENZYMES!

GEORGE

My client, George, a tax lawyer who travels a lot for work, thought he'd never give up drinking coffee every day, or eating sugar, let alone cheese. He'd grown up in the Midwest on a farm and some of his sweetest childhood memories were of homemade apple pie with cheddar cheese.

When he said he'd suffered from such serious colitis most of his life, that it had landed him in the hospital more than once, I suggested he might be sensitive to dairy products.

"Oh, no," he said, "I couldn't live without eating cheese!"

"Well," I countered during our first session," can you imagine what it would be like to live without colitis?"

"No, I can't," he said. "Well, I guess I never thought about it. I've just had it for so long."

I told him, "Diary products and sugar are hard to digest by themselves, but combined together, they're a lethal combination. Would you consider giving them up for two weeks, just to test my theory?"

He answered quickly, "Well, I don't think I can. I'm always traveling for business and you know, it's hard enough just to find time to eat at all!"

After a month without seeing George, he came to see me and said with a resigned sigh, "OK, you win! I had another colitis attack and spent two days in my hotel with spasms that just wouldn't let go. I couldn't figure out why, and then I remembered I'd had a bagel and cream cheese for breakfast, a pastrami sandwich with Swiss cheese for lunch and a cheese plate and fruit for dinner. I thought I was being so good to myself with that fruit and cheese – a light dinner!

"But I was sick as a horse with a bad case of colic – thought maybe they'd have to shoot me or something! I kept thinking about what you'd said – that maybe the dairy is what was getting me. And the sugar, because I usually eat them together. And now I haven't had any dairy or sugar for a week! I was doing much better, and then yesterday I had a cup of coffee and Bam! The pain grabbed me again! So I guess that's gotta go, too."

He sounded like a man who'd just been sentenced to a chain gang. I realized that George's gut might be happy, but his heart was

139

not, so I had an idea. George was a pretty healthy guy, except for his colitis, and I had a hunch he wouldn't need to deprive himself forever of his favorite foods. "George," I said, "take one month and do exactly what you're doing right now. No coffee, no sugar or dairy. And as long as you're at it, I have a few more things for you to let go of. If you're going to clean yourself out, let's go all the way."

When I handed him the 21-day detox diet, he groaned, "Oh Lord," as he perused the "Don't Even Think About it Foods."

"OK, I'll try it," he said. "Right now, I think there's no going back. I already know too much."

George went on to lose 13 pounds along with the pain in his gut and he was thrilled to report that he felt amazing. He even told me it was relatively easy, because he'd been home and his wife had been a supportive cheerleader, as well as captain in the kitchen. When he headed out on the road for two weeks, he emailed me after the first week and said he had stayed away from coffee, sugar and dairy, and had no colitis. He was taking his food enzymes and his powdered greens and then came a moment of truth.

Toward the end of this trip, he was at a business dinner in NYC and he ordered a cup of coffee and a scoop of ice cream. He ate them, and to his absolute delight, there were no repercussions. He went back to his cleaner diet the next day with green tea for breakfast – something he discovered he liked – and his gut stayed calm.

When we spoke, he told me, "I know better than to think I can go back to my old ways of living on cheese sandwiches. But it's great to know that once in a while, I can splurge!"

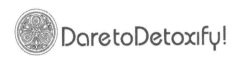

FOOD COMBINING CHART

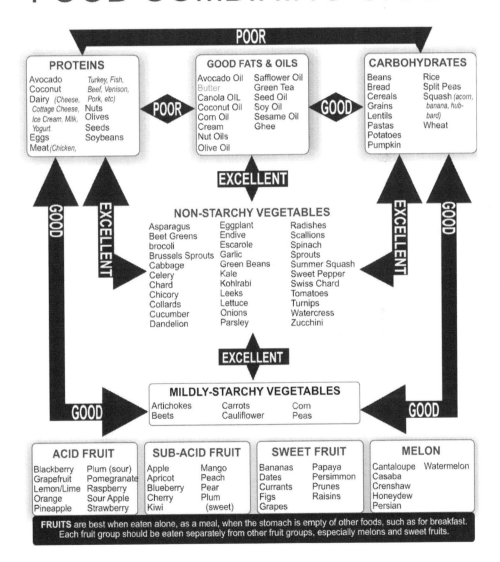

POOR

PROTEINS

Avocado	*Turkey, Fish,*
Coconut	*Beef, Venison,*
Dairy *(Cheese,*	*Pork, etc)*
Cottage Cheese,	Nuts
Ice Cream, Milk,	Olives
Yogurt.	Seeds
Eggs	Soybeans
Meat *(Chicken,*	

POOR

GOOD FATS & OILS

Avocado Oil	Safflower Oil
Butter	Green Tea
Canola OIL	Seed Oil
Coconut Oil	Soy Oil
Corn Oil	Sesame Oil
Cream	Ghee
Nut Oils	
Olive Oil	

GOOD

CARBOHYDRATES

Beans	Rice
Bread	Split Peas
Cereals	Squash *(acorn,*
Grains	*banana, hub-*
Lentils	*bard)*
Pastas	Wheat
Potatoes	
Pumpkin	

EXCELLENT

NON-STARCHY VEGETABLES

Asparagus	Eggplant	Radishes
Beet Greens	Endive	Scallions
brocoli	Escarole	Spinach
Brussels Sprouts	Garlic	Sprouts
Cabbage	Green Beans	Summer Squash
Celery	Kale	Sweet Pepper
Chard	Kohlrabi	Swiss Chard
Chicory	Leeks	Tomatoes
Collards	Lettuce	Turnips
Cucumber	Onions	Watercress
Dandelion	Parsley	Zucchini

GOOD — **EXCELLENT** — **EXCELLENT** — **GOOD**

EXCELLENT

MILDLY-STARCHY VEGETABLES

Artichokes	Carrots	Corn
Beets	Cauliflower	Peas

GOOD — **GOOD**

ACID FRUIT

Blackberry	Plum (sour)
Grapefruit	Pomegranate
Lemon/Lime	Raspberry
Orange	Sour Apple
Pineapple	Strawberry

SUB-ACID FRUIT

Apple	Mango
Apricot	Peach
Blueberry	Pear
Cherry	Plum
Kiwi	(sweet)

SWEET FRUIT

Bananas	Papaya
Dates	Persimmon
Currants	Prunes
Figs	Raisins
Grapes	

MELON

Cantaloupe	Watermelon
Casaba	
Crenshaw	
Honeydew	
Persian	

FRUITS are best when eaten alone, as a meal, when the stomach is empty of other foods, such as for breakfast. Each fruit group should be eaten separately from other fruit groups, especially melons and sweet fruits.

CHAPTER FOURTEEN:
More On Digestion

DIGESTIVE ENZYMES

Enzymes are biocatalysts that make things work faster. They are essential to life! They activate vitamins, minerals, proteins and every other compound in our body. Our digestive enzymes – protease, amylase and lipase, and others – make our digestion work.

Over the years, I have discovered that very few of us make enough digestive enzymes on our own to break down, absorb and efficiently process our food. Even my clients who have great digestion have reported feeling more energy and an improved metabolism when they added food enzymes to their meals. There's a very good reason for this: Cooking destroys enzymes.

That means we have to use our own enzymes to digest everything we eat that is cooked. Dr. Edward Howell, one of America's pioneers in enzymatic research, wrote in his classic book, *Enzyme Nutrition,* that because man evolved on mostly raw food – even raw meat – this contributed 40-60% of its own enzymes to our digestion. That means that our digestive system was designed to use only half of its own energy, our own enzymes, for digestion. Now, however, since many of us eat cooked food, we're using up many more enzymes than

143

we make – if we even have the digestive energy to make them, which many of us don't.

Then our food doesn't digest at all, which creates virtually every digestive disorder there is! That sets the stage for many more degenerative health conditions.

When we don't digest or absorb our food, not only do we get a stomach ache. Our immune system also responds by attacking this partially digested food in our gut. It destroys the food which weakens our immune system and keeps us from getting the nutrients we need. Many allergies are born out of this battle in the intestines.

A lack of enzymes effects the pancreas as well, our blood sugar regulator. Our pancreas has to work double time to make enzymes to digest our cooked food diet, particularly when we eat 8 different foods at one time, from every food group. This puts a huge strain on our pancreas. Then, in the colon, when undigested proteins putrefy, undigested carbohydrates ferment, and undigested fats turn rancid, we get toxicity, not nutrition.

A famous study was conducted from 1932-1942 called the Pottenger Cat Study, with three generations of cats being studied – 900 in all. Dr. Francis Pottenger (the uncle of the doctor I saw when I was 17) took two sets of cats and fed them only raw milk and raw meat. He took three more sets of cats and fed them cooked meat and pasteurized milk. By the end of the second generation, the cats had developed degenerative diseases by mid-life. By the third generation, the cats were developing degenerative diseases early in life, and some were born blind and could not reproduce. Though I've known about this study for 35 years, it just gets more and more relevant as we see serious illness in younger and younger people, as well as infertility. I'm sure when Dr. Pottenger did that study, he didn't realize how prophetic it would be!

But let's get real here. Not everyone is going to eat an all raw diet, and for those who eat meat, that must be cooked. So, how can we get enough enzymes? We can take food enzymes with each of our meals!

Food enzymes, available at the health food store, are made up of each of the enzymes we need for digestion. We recommend our clients take a food enzyme that has hydrochloric acid or *bromelain* if they are eating animal protein. If you try these and your digestive problems worsen – meaning, you experience acid reflux or burning in your throat – you may have a lactic acid condition in your stomach. If so, we suggest you work with a doctor or practitioner who specializes in digestive issues. A company called *Premiere Research* has consultants nationwide who have been very effective in helping clients with this condition.

I suggest you find a food enzyme that is made for digesting every type of food. The only meals you don't need food enzymes for are fruits and raw salads. If you mis-combine foods, a food enzyme can make all the difference in the world as to whether that meal will give you gas and a stomach ache, or move through with ease. Remember Pac-man? I always think of food enzymes as little Pac-men in my stomach, eating everything I didn't chew long enough, or whatever my stomach didn't come up with the energy and digestive juices to turn into liquid. I do believe chewing each bite of food thirty times, like my first grade teacher told me to do, is a virtuous thing, and this chapter on enzymes verifies that! But I've never been a chewer. Maybe that's one reason I don't leave the house without digestive enzymes.

Stress can completely STOP our gut from making enzymes so it isn't smart to eat while you're steaming mad. But so many of my clients have regular business lunches, that if they only ate when the environment was calm, they'd starve! And think about Thanksgiving and Christmas, holidays which make food combining tough. (I'm talking about the buffet here, not just the family dynamics!) This is another place when food enzymes save the day.

SYSTEMIC ENZYMES

You might have heard of "systemic enzymes." These are enzymes that are taken between meals on an empty stomach to help break down the inflammation in our bodies. They can dissolve internal scar tissue and adhesions caused by surgery. For muscle aches and pains, they are more popular in Europe than Advil. Many of our clients have had exceptional results with them. My only caution is that if you've ever had an ulcer, colitis, diverticulitis, or have a very sensitive stomach, they may irritate. You can always try them in small amounts to start. When Allen was in a serious car accident eight years ago, he began taking twelve enzymes a day when he was in the hospital, post-surgery. They were so effective, he never needed a pain pill.

WHEATGRASS JUICE

Ah, wheatgrass, the true staff of life! I first started using wheatgrass in 1980, when I was living in upstate NY with my first husband, David. We had just come home from two years living in Japan, where I'd modeled and was the weather girl on an English language news show. We had left the States filled with energy and strength, having completed two fifteen-day juice fasts in three months. Along with those fasts, we'd been on an organic diet of free-range chicken and fish, vegetables and fruits, and thought this change had surely turned our health problems around permanently.

But it turned out that a year and a half in Japan, living on raw fish, white rice, very few greens and very few vegetables, left us filled with parasites. Our immune systems — which had never been fully flushed or nourished while we lived in Japan — were disintegrating at the speed of a Japanese bullet train! Back to the drawing board. That was when I discovered wheatgrass, living foods, Dr. Ann Wigmore, and the Hippocrates Health Institute.

We bought Dr. Ann's book, *Wheatgrass*, and learned that grass grown from winter wheat berries was one of the most detoxifying and building foods we could put in our bodies. It is more than a food: it is medicine.

Dr. Ann has an inspiring story. Born in Lithuania in 1901, she was abandoned by her parents because she was a sick baby, born premature. Her grandmother, a self-taught natural healer, rescued her. At age 16, never having been allowed to go to school, she could not read or write. Her grandmother coaxed her to come to America where she could get a proper education and live with her parents.

Soon after she arrived, both of her legs were shattered in a horrific automobile accident. The doctors recommended amputation when gangrene set in, but she refused, and against her father's wishes, was sent home. She said, "My homecoming was not a happy one. Neither my father nor my mother would come near me, and only with the help of my uncle would I find something for breakfast."

Ann began eating the diet she had been given by her grandmother: vegetables, grains, nuts, seeds and greens. Remembering what she'd seen her grandmother do, she nibbled on grass and sucked out its juice, and applied poultices of wild greens and grasses to her feet and legs. It took months to heal, but she did, completely. Years later, she ran and successfully completed the Boston Marathon!

She began growing wheat berries indoors, and always an animal lover, she adopted a cancerous monkey and nursed him back to health on a diet of fresh greens, sprouts, fermented seeds and nuts. That's when she knew she was onto something! But she also knew she wasn't going to get people to suck on grass or mow their lawn into a salad, no matter what shape they were in!

At a yard sale one afternoon, she picked up an old cast iron meat grinder, and with a few modifications, this grinder became the first wheatgrass juicer. It was a real turning point because commercial juicers can't extract juice from anything as fibrous as grass. Her innovation made it possible for anyone to grow wheatgrass in their home and extract its juice – something I have been doing daily for over 30 years!

Dr. Ann began delivering juice to ill and elderly people in her Boston neighborhood, and in 1958, moved into an old mansion on Commonwealth Avenue and turned it into "Hippocrates Health Institute." She was not a medical doctor, but many celebrities and researchers flocked to her Institute. Even Yoko Ono purchased a wheatgrass juicer. One researcher, Viktoras Kulvinskas, who was heavily influenced by Dr. Anne's work with wheatgrass juice, wrote a book that caught my attention when I was badly in need of a miracle. He named it *Survival in the 21st Century,* and it was one of the premier books written on natural health and healing.

Wheatgrass juice is nearly identical to human blood, so think of each glass as a blood transfusion. The basic difference is that the hemoglobin (which gives blood its red color) is built around an iron atom, while chlorophyll (which makes plants green) is built around a magnesium atom. So the question arises: Is the body able to substitute iron and rebuild the blood with wheatgrass?

Steve Meyerowitz, also known as "The Sproutman," tells us about an experiment with anemic rabbits in his book, *Wheatgrass, Nature's Finest Medicine*. These rabbits made a rapid return to normal blood count when chlorophyll was administered. It follows that thousands of folks have healed life-threatening illnesses and regenerated compromised organs by incorporating wheatgrass and chlorophyll-rich juices into their diet.

Wheatgrass juice has all known vitamins and minerals, all known proteins and peptides, antioxidants, active enzymes and phytochemicals. It can be absorbed directly through the mucus membranes, and therefore, is excellent for people with digestive problems. I suggest you start your wheatgrass juice intake with an ounce on an empty stomach. This juice is so detoxifying that if it's consumed on top of food, you may experience nausea. I started with one teaspoon a day and now I drink eight ounces every day. Every single day! I feel a rush of energy the moment I swallow it and it sustains me throughout the day. It also lifts my spirits and calms my nervous system, probably due to its high oxygen content and the way it stimulates blood and lymph circulation.

There are many nutritional protocols that can heal serious illnesses. It just happens that wheatgrass therapy and living foods (sprouts and highly digestible greens, consumed raw and juiced) were very effective for me, when I needed a diet that could literally regenerate my tissues and organs. The point is that everyone needs to find what diet works best for them. But the foundation of my living foods diet was the greens, and that hasn't changed. I feel so different on days when I don't get my eight ounces of wheatgrass, because it's such an energy boost.

FREEZE DRIED GREENS: CHLORELLA, BARLEY GRASS, BLUE GREEN ALGAE, SPIRULINA, GREEN MAGMA

When I started using wheatgrass thirty years ago, the shelves at health food stores were not filled with fresh-dried green powders like now. These powders are some of the most transformative foods you can include in your diet. Not to say that adding them means you can eat junk and still be healthy. But they give us on-the-go nutrition, they are extremely alkalizing, and they are packed with nutrients and protein. Greens really are the backbone of any solid nutritional program. I recommend all of the following dried greens: Freeze-dried wheatgrass, Chlorella, barley grass, Green Magma, Blue Green Algae and Spirulina.

Many people find that it's a heck of a lot easier to dump a tablespoon of freeze dried grass or chlorella into their morning smoothie, than it is to buy or squeeze fresh wheatgrass or green juices made of celery, spinach, parsley, sprouts and kale – my favorite all-green combination. If you are healthy and full of energy and just want to reinforce your good luck and your ongoing nutritional program, dried greens are a great addition. If, however, you are healing an illness, struggling with infertility, hoping to regenerate your immune system or re-launch your metabolism, the dried grasses are not alive enough. You'll need fresh juices as many days a week as you can manage, even if you're only taking small amounts.

LAXATIVES

No harsh laxatives please! Besides permanently destroying bowel function with extended use, they cause dehydration and electrolyte loss. If you have constipation, do enemas and get colonics, and use a safe colon cleansing product, such as the kind made by Dr. Richard Schulze (herb-doc.com), that consists of herbs and psyllium seed husks. Or use something gentle that your colonic therapist recommends. I believe that Dr. Schulze makes one of the few safe colon cleansers for children, Intestinal Cleanser #3, which has herbs that actually heal the bowel. I've probably given out 200 bottles of this cleanser to clients with constipated kids or grandparents over the years!

If you have colitis, IBS or diverticulitis, like I did, don't use any bowel cleansing product, no matter what anyone tries to talk you into. They can irritate your colon and cause severe cramping. Drink small amounts of fresh aloe juice daily and sip slippery elm tea. Green juices will also help bowel function, as will castor oil packs, explained below.

All methods considered, colonics are an excellent way to heal an irritable bowel. You may also need to avoid raw salads and eat steamed vegetables. White flour, white sugar, vinegar, coffee and carbonated beverages are disasters for colitis. If you're sensitive, wheat and soy may be disasters for you as well. It would be useful to have what is called an "IGg" blood test for food allergies to determine exactly what the food offenders might be.

CASTOR OIL PACKS

Castor oil packs on the belly are gentle, detoxifying and more effective than you could imagine spreading a bunch of sticky oil on your belly could ever be. Until you remember that everything we put on our skin, we are, in a way, eating! That's right, we're absorbing it through the skin, our largest digestive organ. Edgar Cayce, renowned medical intuitive and psychic of the early 1900s, had many great recipes and tools for healing but castor oil packs are one of his best. They relieve constipation and will detox the liver without harsh side effects (even herbs can have harsh side effects.)

There are many ways I've been taught to do a castor oil pack, and they are all long and complicated. However, they're all effective, so if you're so inclined to research castor oil packs, feel free to do so. I've come up with what I call the *Cheater's Castor Oil Pack*, because it's fast and easy. Therefore, I've found both I and my clients will actually do it. (Don't do it if you're planning a romantic evening, because castor oil is sticky, not slippery, and it doesn't quickly absorb like sesame or almond oil does.)

Before bed, put on an old cotton T-shirt, one you don't mind getting stained. Then slather castor oil (available at health food or drug store) all over your belly, from under your chest to your pubic bone. If you have time, lie with a heating pack over your t-shirt for 20 minutes, so the castor oil can soak in. If not, just let it absorb during the night. By morning, it will assist in promoting a bowel movement. It works really well for kids and babies! I used it with my daughter when she was an infant, and she pooped in half an hour. It does not cause cramps and is safe for those dealing with colitis or other diseases of the colon.

If you want to read an incredible book dedicated to bowel health and cleansing – and you're about to have a lot more bathroom reading time – read Dr. Bernard Jensen's, *Guide to Better Bowel Care*. (Follow it up with something funny, like *The Shit my Father Says* or anything by Annie Lamott. Laughter heals!)

RECTAL IMPLANTS

Another way to introduce electrolytes and probiotics are rectal implants because they allow the electrolytes to be absorbed without upsetting the tummy. These implants, which may contain aloe vera, electrolytes, acidophilus, or chamomile tea are alternative ways to deliver nutrients to the bowel since the colon absorbs anything that goes into the rectum.

Rectal implants are done with syringes that you can buy at the store. Just look for 2-4 ounce "baby ear syringes." Electrolytes are one of the most important nutrients to hydrate the body with after an enema or colonic, but some have vitamin C and can be tough on the stomach. Rectal implants allow the electrolyte to be absorbed without upsetting the tummy.

UNDER THE HOOD – FOR WOMEN ONLY

Having had years of chronic yeast, vaginal and bladder infections, and seeing hundreds of women clients in the same boat, I've learned some natural remedies that really work. It's important to use antibiotics only when you have to. For instance, if you're pregnant and have a bladder infection, your doctor or midwife will want you to take drugs. Otherwise, you might consider the following remedies.

FOR YEAST INFECTIONS

Yeast that resides anywhere in the body lives on sugar, so don't consume any sugar – even fruit or foods that turn into sugar, like simple carbohydrates. Alcohol and fermented foods also aggravate yeast symptoms.

When I have a yeast infection, I use a strong pro-biotic, twice a day. I also take a very effective herbal supplement, that contains pau d'ar-co. But the first thing I do is run to the kitchen to make a garlic tampon.

GARLIC TAMPONS

Garlic cloves can relieve the symptoms of a yeast infection very quickly, when made into a garlic tampon. Ingesting garlic is very helpful, but inserting the clove vaginally is the most effective. However, you can't just insert a raw clove of garlic into your vagina. Because, when it comes time to change cloves, you'll sit there squatting for half an hour trying to get it out, and maybe you'll end up the next day at the Med Center with a story no one will believe! (Except maybe the docs at my local Med Center.)

To make your garlic clove into a tampon, buy the largest bulb of organic garlic you can find. Then take one clove and peel it and cut it at both ends. Next, take a toothpick and stab a hole through the entire clove. Using dental floss (not the minty kind – it's too refreshing), thread the floss through the hole with the toothpick, and tie it at the end. Make sure you've got at least three inches of floss at the bottom. Insert that into your vagina, and change cloves every 6-8 hours.

Finally, the most effective douche I've found is:

One tsp. borax
Five drops tea tree oil
Warm water

I owe the above recipe to Dr. Robert Pottenger, the doctor who saved my life when I was a teenager. When he told me to go out and buy 20 Mule Team Borax for a vaginal infection, I thought he was nuts! But it works.

Apple cider vinegar also makes an excellent douche. But be sure to wear all-cotton undies! Even yoga pants have spandex in them, so while the infection is still active, an unnatural fiber will keep the air from flowing and trap the bacteria. Let your vagina breathe.

BLADDER INFECTIONS

Bladder infections can be dangerous, because they can become kidney infections. You can do a home test for them, and if you are testing positive for both leukocytes and nitrates, you should contact your doctor who will want to test you as well. He or she will decide if you have time to try a natural remedy or not.

If you don't test positive for a bladder infection, but have the symptoms of one – pain when urinating, frequent urination and discomfort in the abdomen – you can try an herbal remedy. The most effective one I've found is Dr. Richard Schulze's Kidney/Bladder tincture, taken every three hours. It contains uva ursi and other herbs that clean and detoxify the bladder and kidneys. Along with that, I use a cranberry concentrate in pill form, and D Mannose powder, all available at your health food store. Step up the Vitamin D3 as well.

CHAPTER FIFTEEN
Say Good-Bye to "Normal!"

You don't really need me to tell you that sugar, caffeine, and junk food is going to make you sick, depressed, fat and cranky. I hope you've learned something from reading this book, but if you're like most of my clients and have been around the block once or twice, you've heard at least some of this before! You know it makes sense or you wouldn't have bought the book. But your struggle is – doing it!! Years ago, my former husband, Kenny, wrote, "The gates of hell are locked from the inside," and it's a line most of us can relate to.

Everyone wants the secret to self discipline, the ability to consistently choose salads and veggies over processed mac and cheese. We all want to eat these healthy foods every single day without suffering, or feeling so deprived that the moment we finally feel fantastic, when those jeans fit and the migraines are gone, we feel an uncontrollable urge to pig out on pizza! As a "reward!"

The key to a healthy and beautiful body is not in the fine print. That's the stuff that most diet books are made of, and many authors have made a mint, coming up with gimmicks that make it appear as though substituting brown rice for white, or tofu for beef, or eating only purple foods for a month, will save your soul and ass. Forget it!

157

The key to radical health is activating your own, individual awareness as to what makes your body feel good and run efficiently. Then you have to find the key to surrender to eating that way on order to give yourself day-in and day-out health and vitality.

This is not about what makes our mouths happy because most of that is habit. It isn't what our mom fed us as a kid or what looks "normal" at a business dinner. Our society's "*normal*" in anything – especially mainstream food – is death to health and happiness. The only useful thing to do with "mainstream food" is to make a poster of everything that stereotypically can be classified under that heading and take it out into the backyard and burn it!!

You need to understand that sheer willpower will not work for the long haul. It barely works for the itty bitty short haul. The only way that this or any other lifestyle change works is for it to feel as *natural* as breathing. That will take time. Change doesn't come overnight. The ritual of coffee and a Danish has to be replaced by an equally luscious treat, with luscious company. True Detox is not only about getting toxins out of your body, but getting poisonous and self-sabotaging behavior out of your mind, out of your daily habits, and out of your life.

In the end, no matter how much you know, the most challenging part of detoxing is doing it. But it is possible to do, especially if you can find a friend, a detox partner or a mate, to do it with you. What's working against you here – until you get it working for you – is the ancient very human desire to be part of the group, It is our ancestral roots in tribes and community.

No matter how much physical pain someone is in, I've discovered that the most painful thing for most of my clients is the idea of not participating in the rituals of their families and circle of friends – and

158

most of these rituals involve food. People die over this loyalty every day. It's so deeply ingrained in us that most of us don't even know why we cave in and eat that donut. We think it's because we're weak and we're wracked with shame and guilt when we "go off the wagon." God only knows how toxic that shame and guilt is – worse than the hydrogenated fats and sugars. But the truth is that we're not weak. Most of us just want desperately to belong. From the beginning of time, being exiled was a fate worse than death or torture, and we all carry that cellular memory. So how can you turn down a piece of cake if a little voice in your head says, "Aah, that cake means I'm part of the tribe!"

It's time to change that, as individuals, as parents, as partners. We need to be bold enough and brave enough to re-invent every single one of our rituals, so that healthy choices are synonymous with being loved, included and desired. We can't do this alone. We need to do it in groups, with our mates and where we work. Just as some of us have had to reframe what it means to be in a healthy relationship, we must do the same with food.

If you've been a rebel – a non-conformist who became a cheese-loving vegetarian at the age of 12, or chose carrot juice over coffee as a point of pride – there are changes for you to make, as well. I am you, so I know all about the trap of the rebel. When you rebel against something, you skip right over your natural instincts. You're not in touch with your intuition. You're not doing what's right for you. You're just determined to *not* do what the other person is doing. It's not freedom – it is its own jail. I know from personal experience how important it is to stay in touch with my body's dietary needs, which have changed over the years, and will continue to change. Self-preservation — being a warrior for one's true needs — does not come easy for many of us!

159

There are many ways to activate your own self-preserver. Some of my clients have found that joining Food Anonymous was very helpful, and going to meetings gave them a cheering squad and group to whom to be accountable. Yoga allows the body and mind to align in a way that supports massive changes, all the way from your head to your toes. It is detoxifying, regenerative and energizing. Hypnotherapy, EMDR, acupuncture and bio-feedback are all excellent for healing the sources of your self-sabotage, especially when it comes to bucking your core beliefs about yourself.

Do you deserve to be healthy, happy and beautiful? Are you stuffing crap in your mouth because you hate your job or you're lonely? Is food your substitute for a lover and playmate? I have learned so much from the educational programs of David deAngelo (for men) and Rori Raye and Christian Carter (for women, both available through the net on CD or DVD), and of Gay and Kathlyn Hendricks, on relationship and creating commitment: Commitment to one's self first, and then, a lasting and exciting, love and marriage. If you eat because you struggle with loneliness and relationship issues (including the one with yourself) check out their work!

For kids and teenagers, my sister, Susan Cooper, and her partner, June Salin, created *The Manadoob* an internationally recognized, award-winning self-esteem program for kids, with a book and workbook to help children of all ages get in touch with and talk about tough feelings and experiences like loss, grief, rage, divorce and death. The book comes with stones – somewhat like Runes – that kids can hold in their hands, and a bracelet that says, "I believe!" Can you imagine what it would have been like for you as a child, if you had been able to feel what you felt and express it to a compassionate, loving adult?

The farther we stray from the lifestyle of our parents, our friends and extended family, the more uncomfortable we may feel when we're initiating a program as life-changing as detoxification. If we can use the discomfort we feel when we begin this program – the knot in our stomach, the fog in our brains, the cloudiness that crosses our eyes and the pressure in our chests – to measure just how courageous we are and how far we've come to be ready, willing and able to give ourselves the life we were meant to live, and the body we were meant to live in – then, we have the strength and patience to breathe through any bumps in the road.

The Hoffman Process is an incredible one-week training in San Francisco that helps us rip apart our childhood programming and determine what beliefs are truly ours, and what might belong to our mom or dad. This is very helpful when it comes to re-wiring our dietary code. During the Process, you write, you cry, you scream and re-invent your life. I recommend it to everyone. I was lucky enough to do it when I was 24 and it was life-saving and life-changing.

Another life saving and life-changing tool is the detox partner I mentioned earlier – a friend, a mate, a relative who will grocery shop with you, answer the phone when you find yourself driving to the AM/PM to buy French fries and ice cream at 1 am, and someone who thinks it's hilarious that your enema bag broke just before the in-laws arrived. When we're leaving old habits behind and we're leaping blindly towards a new world and a new version of ourselves, it helps to have a safety net. I will be forever indebted to all those who have been there for me. I believe I would not be here without them.

MAKE IT YOUR OWN

Allen, Anita and I experimented with dozens of protocols over many years in order to come up with a diet and cleansing program that works for us. And each of our programs is different. Yours will be, too. There is no ONE WAY. Don't let anyone tell you that their way is the only way! Some people feel best eating all raw. Others feel best eating some clean meat. You won't know how your body runs most efficiently until all the crap is out of it. And since the only thing we can count on in life is change, our optimal diet will change, too. Having the tools of detoxification will allow you to be so tuned in to your body's needs, you'll actually know if you need more protein or more carbohydrates. You will be in touch with your gut instincts, because after a thorough detoxification, you will feel clean, clear, light and bursting with natural optimism and joy. That is everyone's birthright!

Though I became involved in detox to save my life, as Allen did for Anita, I continued on my journey of regular detox cleanses to enhance and maintain a strong quality of life. I eat the way I do, and avail myself of other healing modalities so that I can live, love and have the most fun possible. Otherwise, really, what's the point?! Mary Oliver, one of my favorite poets, said that there is one question to ask: "What do you plan to do with your one wild and precious life?" I dare you to answer that question as boldly as you can...and I wish for you all the energy you deserve to accomplish all your dreams...

Yours in radical health and wild happiness,

Julia

To Spirit, to all the energy in the universe,

To the storms that rage within me and outside of me

To the nights that at times seem endless

And the dawn that I vow to meet with equanimity and faith

Please fill me with the courage to dream,

To reclaim my innocent heart and my tender, fierce

Devotion to live an extraordinary life.

Please give me the courage to sit with my demons,

To invite them into the room rather than plot

Their assasination,

Knowing and trusting they will gladly turn from toxic

To benign as I accept that they no longer have

Their hands around my neck.

Let them speak…

Let them writhe…

Let them educate me about my past so that my present may be

Born out of their ashes,

Out of their clouds, out of their waste, out of my pain…

I am never alone…

I am held by Spirit and the wisdom of my beating heart

I am rich in friendship and community,

I do not hesitate to ask for or give support…

Today I dare to take my life into my own hands,

And live it as loudly as I can!

Bibiography

1) The Second Brain, by Michael D. Gershon, M.D.

2) Dr. Jenson's Guide to Better Bowel Care, by Dr. Bernard Jenson

3) Breakthrough, by Suzanne Sommers

4) The Detox Strategy, by Brenda Watson

5) Never Be Sick Again, by Raymond Francis, M.Sc.

6) Cleanse and Purify Thyself, Volume 1, by Richard Anderson, ND, NMD

7) Inside Poop, by Scott W. Webb

8) Cleansing Made Simple, by Cheryl Townsley, ND

9) The Detox Book, by Bruce Fife, ND

10) The Raw Food Detox Diet, by Natalia Rose

11) The Human Colon, By William Grace, Stewart Wold and Harold G. Wolf

12) Jumping for Health, by Dr. Morton Walker

13) Heal from the Inside Out, by Reul Ari

14) Always Look Out for Number Two, by Galina Imrie

15) Fit for Life, by Harvey and Marilyn Diamond

16) Colon Health, by Dr. Norman Walker

17) The Fertility Solution, by Niravi Payne

18) Heal and Cleanse Thyself, Volume 2, by Richard Anderson, ND, NMD

19) Wheatgrass, By Ann Wigmore

20) Wheatgrass, Nature's Finest Medicine, by Steve Meyerowitz

21) There Are No Incurable Diseases, by Dr. Richard Schulze

22) The Gerson Therapy, by Charlotte Gerson and Morton Walker, DPM

23) Healing and Detoxification by Dr. Sidney MacDonald Baker, M.D.

24) Digestive Wellness, By Elizabeth Lipski, PhD, CCN

25) Natural Detoxification, by Jacqueline Krohn, M.D.

26) Balancing the Body's ph, with Kangen Water, by Joan Vandergriff, ND

(27) Overcoming The Acid Crisis, by Martha M. Christy

(28) Detoxification, Volume 2, by Dr. Richard Schulze

(29) Optimal Health for Longevity, by Dr. Brian Clement

Glossary Of Terms

DETOXIFICATION

In this book, detoxification refers to the removal of environmental, physical, emotional and pharmaceutical toxins from the body. These kinds of seasonal cleansings can benefit us all by helping our bodies eliminate the toxins from food sources and our environment that have become trapped in our bodies.

COLONIC

A colonic is a painless, safe and effective method of cleansing the colon – the last six feet of the large intestine which can hold from five to twenty pounds of waste at any given time. The bottom line is that if our colons aren't healthy, we're not healthy. Elvis died, not of a drug overdose or heart failure, but rather of an impacted colon – fifty pounds, to be exact!

When the colon is not completely empty, the liver, gall bladder and kidneys don't release toxins. In the compromised and polluted environment in which we live, our organs of elimination are working over-time. Because neurotoxins (poisons that effect the brain and nervous system) are accessed through the colon, colonics can help relieve headaches and depression.

LYMPH MASSAGE

Lymph is the interstitial fluid that comprises 70-80% of the liquid in our bodies, making up a substantial portion of our cardiovascular circulatory system. A lymph massage is a gentle technique which assists in moving the lymph out of the tissue and back to the bloodstream, transporting fat, proteins, hormones and nutrients throughout the body. Lymph is as important as our blood, yet it is often totally neglected and misunderstood. It is not pumped by the heart like blood is. Rather, it must be activated by massage, exercise and dry skin brushing. When it gets sluggish, it becomes a cesspool of viruses, bacteria and even cancer cells. Cleansing this system is a key to the healing and strength of not only our hearts, but also our immune systems, our endocrine systems (hormones and adrenal function) and our ability to eliminate inflammation, which the AMA has recently recognized as a major cause of disease.

pH

pH is a term that defines the acid/alkaline balance of our bodies. In a healthy person, the numbers should range between 6.4 and 7.4. You can test your own urine and saliva with strips purchased at a health food or drug store. Always remember that a balanced pH is a necessary ingredient for optimum health and vitality!

Resources:

Julia Loggins at

www.DARETODETOXIFY.com

The Clinic for Drugless Therapy,

Julia Loggins and Wesley Roe

120 1/2 W. Mission Street,

Santa Barbara, CA 93103

805-563-0062

Santa Barbara, CA

Santa Barbara Center for Lymphatic Health

www.lymphatichealth.com

214 1/2 De La Guerra Street

Santa Barbara, CA 93101

805-962-1882

American Health Institute

Dr. Michael Galitzer and Dr. Janet Hranicky

12381 Wilshire Blvd., Suite 102

Los Angeles, CA

310-820-6042

1-800-392-2623

American Academy For the Advancement of Medicine

ACAM.com

Hippocrates Health Institute

www.hippocratesinst.org

1465 Skees Rd.

West Palm Beach, FL 33411

561-471-8876

The MANADOOB.com

www.manadoob.com

International Assocation of Colon Therapists

www.i-act.org

READY TO TAKE YOUR CLEANSING TO A
WHOLE NEW LEVEL ?

Julia Loggins and Wesley Roe welcome you to our clinic in beautiful Santa Barbara!! We are open six days a week, and we are excited to facilitate your cleansing and detoxification. Dare to dump that tired, stressed out and toxic body, and transform it into an unstoppable, lean and energized machine! The time is now, Your health is your most valuable asset.

Experience The Santa Barbara 3-Day, 7-Day or 14-Day Cleansing Program, personally designed for your individual needs, with Santa Barbara's most esteemed wellness counselors. Stay in one of Santa Barbara's lovely inns, hotels or bed and breakfasts, and give yourself the vacation of a lifetime. Experience the extraordinary lightness that comes from letting go of a lifetime of toxicity....the program includes a personally designed detox diet, colonic hydrotherapy, lymphatic drainage, physical therapy/IMT (a cutting edge form of physical therapy, especially effective for those with autoimmune challenges), chiropractic and/or acupuncture treatments, as needed.

We Offer:

Individually Designed Cleansing Programs
3-day, 7-day or 14-day

Private Consultations

Lifestyle support for transitional and detoxification diets

Travel support for busy professionals

Colon Hydrotherapy

Our favorite products and supplements will be available on our website, daretodetoxify.com....so visit us with all your specific detoxification needs and download a free food combining chart!

Referrals for detoxification experts all over the country are also available by contacting us on our website. No matter where you live, we'd love to hear from you!

Visit us at The Clinic for Drugless Therapy!

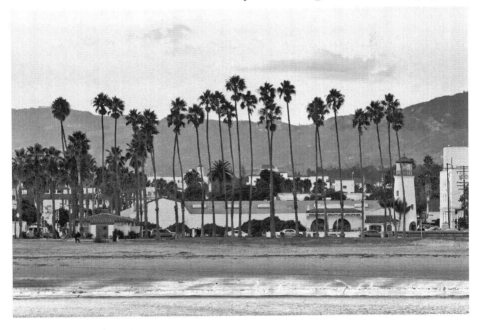

The Clinic For Drugless Therapy
120 1/2 W. Mission
Santa Barbara, CA 93101
805.563.0062
DaretoDetoxify.com

16022740R00099

Made in the USA
San Bernardino, CA
15 October 2014